Dr. Chi's Method

of

FINGERNAIL

and

TONGUE DIAGNOSIS

How to use teethmarks and Lunulae diagnosis for the prevention of Cancer, heart disease, hormones, and digestive problems.

CHi

TSU-TSAIR CHI N.M.D, Ph.D

ISBN 0-9657847-9-7

Printed in U.S.A.

Preface

Returning to The Roots of Medicine

Medicine and health care are returning to their roots, especially here in the United States. While "natural medicine" has co-existed with "Western Style" medicine in many areas of our world, it has been forced 'underground' in the United States (and much of the world which considers itself civilized) for most of the 20th century.

Fortunately, the limitations of "high-tech", drug and surgery-intensive health care are being realized both here and abroad. While sometimes lifesaving in emergency situations, drugs and surgery have little to offer for longer-term, chronic illness, or for prevention of disease before it happens. "Western medicine" is also enormously expensive, and many families and governments can no longer afford it!

So the newspapers, television, radio, books and magazines are full of "natural healing", vitamins, minerals, herbs and botanical remedies, acupuncture, homeopathy, Qi gong, and many other natural techniques... and those of us who didn't know are rapidly learning their value. Even "orthodox physicians" are taking an interest.

But before healing comes diagnosis, "Western medicine" has too frequently made diagnosis a high-tech, laboratory-intensive, x-ray and CAT-scan affair, as expensive as high-tech treatment. Many older physicians, while admiring the occasional stunning finding of a tiny tumor on an MRI, still deplore the marked decline in the teaching of "hands-on", observation-based physical diagnosis skills in today's "modern" medical schools.

Along with the 'roaring renaissance' in natural treatments

comes a quieter but equally important trend; the re-emergence of interest in "hands-on" physical diagnosis, using close observation of the 'patient' and extensive knowledge of body systems in health and disease. Applied kinesiology", foot reflexology, iridology, and intuitive methods of diagnosis are attracting more interest, and are slowly emerging from the "far fringes" of diagnostic techniques.

Other cultures have their methods, too, and we are learning that there may be value in methods "not invented here", especially if they have a several thousand year old tradition, as do many Chinese and Ayurvedic (Indian) techniques. Would people likely as intelligent as we have used there methods for those thousands of years if there were nothing at all to them?

I have been quite ignorant of tongue and fingernail diagnosis (except that they existed), and was surprised when Dr. Chi asked me to write this forward to this book about them. Having read it through, I can see I once again have something to learn, but it's something that will help me greatly in helping the people with whom I work each day at Tahoma Clinic. Perhaps that was Dr. Chi's point....if so, I am grateful, and if not, I am happy to have a page or two to write for you in the book of an accomplished master of the art of physical diagnosis, the beginning and "root"of good medicine in any century.

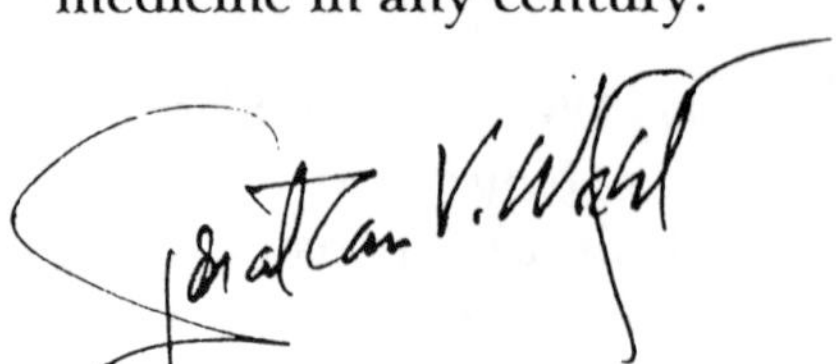

Jonathan v. Wright, M.D.
Tahoma Clinic
Kent, Washington
U.S.A.

Preface

It has been my pleasure to be acquainted with Dr. Tsu-Tsair Chi for the last four years. I have been able to review his work and have found it to be most intriguing. Since 1976, I have been personally involved with Chinese medicine, molecular design, evaluation of creative thought and application.

I am most impressed with Dr. Chi's approach to physical diagnosis. However, his ability to transform Chinese Medicines into therapeutic agents that are accepted within the confines of Western mentality is of equal importance. Products such as water soluble herbal tablets and natural powders that instantly dissolve in liquid are the results of the bridge between the methods of the east and those of the west that Dr. Chi has admirably built.

Clearly, Dr. Chi's research and work merits the respect of all physicians. Those who employ his techniques will vastly enhance their diagnostic prowess without resorting to more invasive forms of technology. I am grateful to have encountered these techniques and hope that my colleagues will find them to be equally beneficial to their practice.

Sincerely,

Morris A. Mann, M.D.

CONTENTS

INTRODUCTION

The technique for fingernail and tongue diagnosis saw its development over thousands of years, resulting in a methodology that is so astutely precise and so natural that it may be well-described as an enlightened art form. Eastern doctors have used much of it successfully throughout the generations, and it is this tradition that allows its type of diagnosis to hold its place as both an excellent medical tool and an indelible mark of our culture. My own father was a doctor for forty-five years, and I myself have had eighteen years of experience in the field. Together we have been able to combine both eastern and western methodologies through the generations to create a unique program in physical diagnosis. Both patients and doctors alike have been urging me to publish some of this valuable information, and I hope this book will serve as both an innovative guide to medical diagnosis and a carefully planned bridge to bring together two schools of thought, culminating in an advanced look at the future of medicine and preventative diagnosis based on physical markers. And unlike most other handbooks on Chinese medicine which will tell you to forget everything you learned about Western medicine and start over with a whole new system, my approach will allow you to combine what you already know with knowledge in Asian medicine to achieve the best results.

Throughout the years, I have had the opportunity to see many patients and have managed to compile the clinical data of over 10,000 cancer patients from around the world.

Interestingly, there appeared to be two major markers on the body that have been shown to be correlative to these patients' conditions. Using these two common markers, I have been able to categorize these patients into eight different symptomatic categories pinpointing the origins of their conditions. Of these categories, one represents the characteristics of a healthy person, while the other seven represent different problematic situations that are possible in people.

I have written this book, in part, in response to the large demand of people who wish to learn more about this cultural and family treasure. From the mention of my techniques in an October 1996 Scientific American article to countless phone calls to our office in Anaheim, the public is becoming increasingly interested in my diagnostic methods, and I hope this will help everyone to better understand what I have been doing for years.

Readers should note that diseases do not always have easily detectable causes and symptoms. In some cases the same disease may be found to give quite different symptoms among people. Similarly, the same symptoms in people can be caused by quite different diseases. Thus, to arrive at an accurate diagnosis is often a difficult task. A mere one or two self-exams is not always sufficient for proper diagnosis. Often one needs to use detailed, frequent analyses to get a subjective determination. And when the condition shows itself to be severe, a physician must be seen immediately. Early detection of problems allow for early treatment and a better chance of healing, but treatment is a necessary component that cannot be put off lest it lead to worse, or even irremediable situations.

Finally, I would like to thank my family, Cheryl, Jennifer, and Shirley for helping me complete this work. Without their help, support, and dedication, this would not have been possible. I would also like to express my deepest gratitude to my father, Dr. Kui-Chen Chi, for his knowledge and guidance.

Tsu-Tsair Chi, N.D., Ph.D.
Anaheim, January 1997

Introduction to Fingernail and Tongue Analysis

Throughout history, doctors have always been given the sole responsibility of diagnosing people for health problems. However, as society advances and medicine and science progress, the mentality of the public changes also. People have learned the importance of early diagnosis, and one of the major methods of early diagnosis is regular self-examination. Medical statistics show that, of the cases of breast adenocarcinomas, about 95% of patients detected the problem themselves by self-examination and the finding of lumps in their breasts. Only about 5% of cases are diagnosed by doctors. The number of women who detected the cancers themselves outnumber doctor diagnoses by a factor of 18, showing the relevance and importance of the knowledge involved in self-examination.

Many other diseases besides breast cancer can be self-diagnosed, and if every family knew the basics of self-diagnosis, then the important task of early detection leading to early treatment can finally be carried out. The benefits of early detection are clear and many, and thus there is no need to discuss them at this point.

Because of all this, we feel that a widespread familiarization with the methods of self-diagnosis is necessary. Everyone needs to know, besides this, how to take preventative steps toward the improvement of a condition that could lead to disease. This has become the role of doctors in today's world of growing populations and health concerns, to not only diagnose and treat, but to teach others the methods of preventative and early self-diagnosis.

The most widely accepted method of diagnosis by far in the Eastern culture is the tongue diagnosis, and is especially used in Chinese medicine, along with pulse diagnosis. Fingernail diagnosis, ear diagnosis, foot reflexology and acupressure have also been used in the past. Ear diagnosis, however, is difficult to implement since the telling physical marks on the ear are much more subtle and not as prominent as tongue or fingernail physical markers. Pulse diagnosis is also difficult to carry out accurately since the pulse is often hard to hear, and the differences in pulse that correspond to differences in bodily function and health and therefore much harder to ascertain.

So why have I chosen instead to use the fingernails and tongue to do quick and accurate readings of organ function? The fingernails have the capacity to show very openly detectable characteristics that correspond to organ function and bodily health. This physical clarity of nail markers allow the fingernails to accurately show the condition of the body in a clear and easily seen way. However, since a full nail usually takes between 6-8 months in adults to grow out, their markers are generally slow to appear and disappear as the bodily condition changes. The tongue, however, regenerates its entire topmost epithelial layer every 3 days. This fast rate of regrowth allows for immediate detection of problems, faster than any other form of physical diagnosis. These two methods combined together can work to produce precise results from both a chronic disease standpoint and an acute one, through comparing the findings of either method. For instance, a chronic disease would show severe correlating physical markers on *both* the tongue and fingernail, while a minor or acute disease would only show up in the tongue. Thus, it is my belief that both the tongue AND fingernail diagnostic methods should be introduced to everyone, and I hope that this combination can stir discussion among professionals and trigger input from these groups.

This type of analysis is very useful in that doctors will be able to discern the patient's problem with 80% accuracy even before any blood tests, hair analyses, or urinalyses results come back from the lab. This type of analysis can direct the doctor's attention to one of the 5 major areas of the body, and the exact problem can be further pinpointed after that by the physician. Thus, doctors can get a good idea of what their patient's problem is without having to search blindly using exploratory techniques, and perhaps even start treatment early enough to stave off future complications. For patients, this can prove quite advantageous in terms of saving money in unnecessary laboratory fees.

The two major markers that are used in this type of analysis to identify bodily problems are: A) the fingernails, and B) the tongue. By looking at either one or both of these bodily markers, we can direct the problem to one (or more) of the 5 different important organ areas of the human system, as prescribed by the ancient Chinese method: the liver, the heart, the spleen, the lung, and the kidney.

About the 5 systems

The Chinese have relied on a system represented by the interconnections between the 5 main organs of the body for thousands of years. These different systems correlate to the 5 main traditional "elements" of the ancient Chinese system: wood, fire, earth, metal, and water (See Chart A). These were the elements that were believed to be in existence in the heavens during the time before the invention of scientific apparati, before the advancement of the understanding of the natural world, yet they are remarkably accurate when translated into medical views.

In the 5-system methodology, the liver system represents the area of bodily detoxification. The area of the heart represents the circulatory system and the mental-psychological welfare of the person. The spleen area represents the blood-producing components of the body, as well as the immune system and the digestive system. The lung area represents the respiratory and lymphatic systems, and the kidney area represents the reproductive, endocrine and excretory systems.

Following the 5-system diagram, the solid arrows that form a star on the diagram represent the interconnection of the different organ systems. For instance, a healthy liver system will lead to a healthy spleen as well, and vice versa. Similarly, if the kidney is weak, then that in turn leads to a weakness in the heart. Based on this knowledge, it can be seen that problems of the lung may often be associated to heart trouble, and may not be isolated to respiratory conditions alone. Someone with poor kidney function may be derive the problem from weakness or dysfunction of the spleen, as can be seen by the arrow leading from the spleen to the kidney. This shows that problems of the spleen can, by flow of systems, cause problems in the kidneys. Similar conclusions can be drawn with the other systems connected

5 SYSTEMS

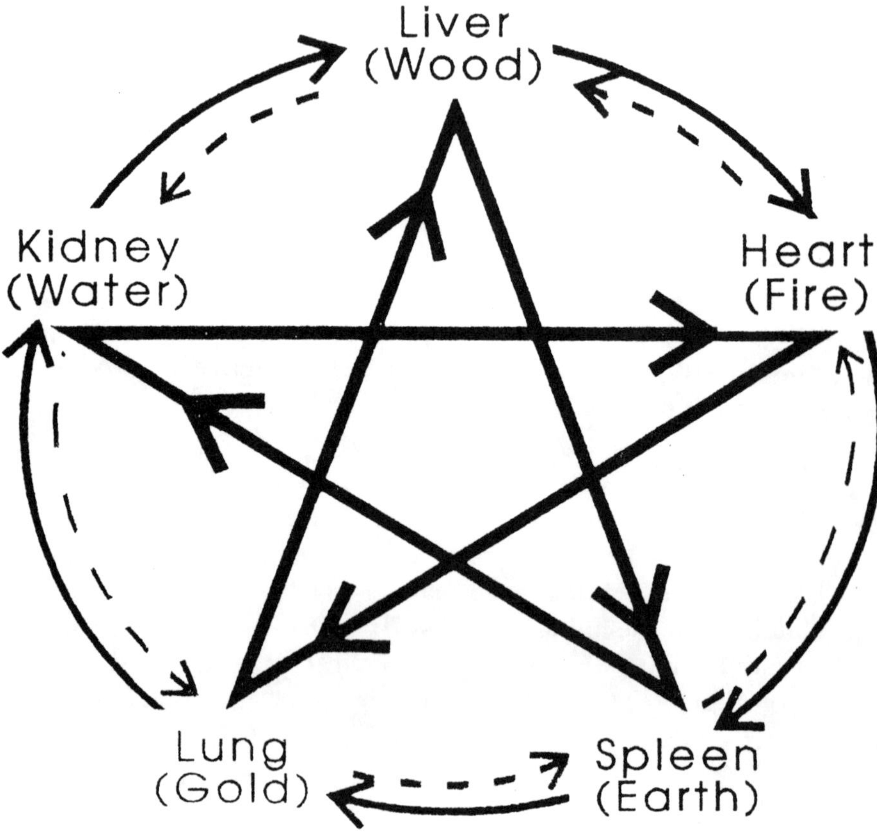

Chart A

by the arrows as well.

The circular solid and broken-line arrows connecting adjacent systems represent the equilibrium between the systems. If a certain system is too strong, it will be balanced by weaker adjacent systems. For instance, if the lung system is too strong, then the kidney and the spleen, being adjacent to it on the diagram, will be weaker. This is correlative to the "hot-cold" mixed description, where the Yin and Yang of the body are unbalanced, resulting in the mixed symptoms of the patient. For instance, an overly active kidney can oftentimes be "balanced out" by poor liver or lung function. These types of patients commonly get illnesses, especially colds, and have a higher mortality rate when it comes to severe disorders.

In the next section we shall discuss how to diagnose the fingernails as the first step in the combined self-diagnostic method I have developed. Part II will be dedicated to diagnosing the tongue as the next crucial component of self-diagnosis. Part III will focus on other methods of self-diagnosis, including eye and skin tests, that will work to confirm the results of the fingernail and tongue diagnosis.

Part I

Fingernail Diagnosis

1

Overview of the Fingernail Diagnosis

A good practitioner should be able to tell if a patient's organs are healthy or weak just by looking at the appearance of her nails. Because hands are the part of the body that require the most flexibility and facultative potential for movement, they are able to reflect a person's physical and spiritual condition. Nails never finish their cycle of growth and, thus, are an accurate record of a person's systemic and physical situation.

Nails are the transfer point for all nutrients in the body. Blood runs through these specific points, which are the meridian points of the body. Many physical deficiencies can be seen in the appearance of the nails. If in good health, the nails will be shiny in luster, pink colored and transparent, with an even, smooth arch. If one maintains a proper diet, they are quite healthy.

Although there are many different systems in the body to speak of, my family has always referred to several specific ones that correlate to each fingernail. Thus, the five fingernails on each hand refer to a certain part of the body:

The thumbnail-

The thumbnail reflects the condition of the brain, the

excretory system, and the reproductive system. For instance, if the thumb is the only nail that presents a problem, then this person may have a localized malady.

The index fingernail-
This nail reflects the condition of the liver, gall bladder, and the nervous system. If the index finger is brittle and of a greyish yellow or a dark green color, and is the only finger that presents a problem, then this person is easily prone to liver, gall bladder, or nervous system maladies.

The middle fingernail-
If the middle fingernail is the only nail that presents a problem, then this is generally not a good sign. If the middle fingernail is abnormal, then this patient has a heat and circulatory problem.

The ring fingernail-
The ring fingernail has, throughout ancient times, been related to reproductive organ function, along with the body's hormonal balance to a certain degree.

The pinkie finger-
The condition and appearance of this fingernail reflects the condition of the digestive system and gastro-intestinal tract, including the stomach, intestines, and colon.

Generally, nails should have a hard, epithelial cornea layer. Hardness of the nails can also say a lot about the patient's physical situation. A patient who has overly soft nails has very sensitive nerves and is suffering from poor nutrition. Thin, soft nails can also refer to a calcium deficiency. Nails that appear brittle and are plagued with large cracks signify that the patient suffers from malnutrition and adrenal gland problems. Brittle nails also signify problems in the patient's excretory and reproductive systems. Healthy people often have nails that can be characterized as being elastic and strong. Healthy nails are also translucent in color, showing a pink hue with a smooth, even face and a slight shine. Healthy nails should be somewhat elastic and should be of the correct thickness. The correct amount of thickness is 0.5-0.75 mm. Nails grow faster in the summer and on male youths and adults than in women.

One thing that should be noted first off when performing a fingernail analysis is the consistency of the nails overall, and their general appearance. Many basic, important facts can be drawn from this kind of general diagnosis. Shriveled, atrophied, or thin nails, for instance, signify that the patient is malnourished and may often experience cramps in his extremities. Nails which are easily broken at short lengths could be due to tinea, athlete's foot, or ringworm caused by trichophyton, which is a difficult fungal infection to treat. Heat rash and prickly heat can also cause tinea, which is also very difficult to cure. Flesh that separates from the nail, leaving the nail with a yellow appearance could be a sign that the patient is suffering from dermatitis or anemia. If the nail and the flesh have separated so that only part of the nail is connected to the flesh, then this person has eczema.

If a patient's nails become rough and yellow and if the nail-growth diminishes its speed , then this person may be suffering from diabetes, heart disease, or poor capillary circulation. If the matrix of the nails is experiencing atrophic changes such as discoloration or sudden swelling, this may be due to lupus (hardened skin). Nails that conform to the above symptoms, as well as matrix atrophy, signify that the patient has diabetes.

If nails are brittle, or if they can be flexed and bent too easily, then bones may be similarly weak. Based on kidney hormones, if the bone breaks, calcium needs to be quickly deposited. This way, kidney hormones can replenish their mineral deposits more quickly. Brittle nails indicate that the kidney is in bad condition and that blood supply to nails are not enough to bring enough nutrition. Anemia, chemotherapy, or poor blood circulation may have an after--effect that is apparent in the nails which will result in dull, weak nails that are not elastic but brittle, thus breaking easily.

Lastly, and before we begin our detailed journey into fingernail analysis, let me suggest following along the next few chapters with my diagnostic kit, a turntable wheel designed for easy clarification of fingernail condition. It may prove helpful in the general schema to look at this kit while reading the chapters.

2

NAIL SHAPE and CURVATURE

The face of the nail, which should be proportional to the hands and the rest of the body, can well reveal how the body is functioning. For instance, if a patient has short nails, then she should proportionately have short fingers. The nails of a patient should not deviate notably from each other. They should be arched in a slightly curving structure, transparent to reveal the pink flesh beneath, and normal in size. If a patient has short, square-shaped nails instead, then she has a hyper-excitable condition. If the nails are short to a certain level and very small, then the patient may have heart disease. If the nails are too long, then the patient may have respiratory problems. A patient who has parallel vertical lines on the thumbnail shows signs of a kidney problem that may derive from old age (Fig. 1-a, Pic. 1-a). If this appearance is conspicuous, on all the nails, and the nails have already begun to darken, then the patient is suffering from a respiratory problem which may be caused by what is called a mineral insemination problem (Pic. 1-b, c). What this means is that the body's needed trace elements are not being absorbed properly, and either they are not getting enough of these vital minerals, or their bodies are not using them up correctly. Basically, all minerals that we ingest either through food or supplements is in its unreactive and thus unusable form. For our bodies to be able to use these minerals, they must be in a charged, or ionized form, undergoing an energy-expending process. This bioenergy is missing from our natural consumption of sun rays due to carbon dioxide and moisture absorption. However, this phenomenon can be prevented by using the mineral infrared device (See Appendix A on MIT and also *Dr. Chi's Guide to Health with Mineral Frequency and Herbs*.) An example of this can be seen in hemoglobin, the oxygen-carrying substance in our blood. Hemoglobin has a protein component called porphyrin, which is bound to positively charged iron before it can be active. However, the iron that we ingest is in its uncharged form, and thus it takes an amount of energy to remove some electrons (thus leaving a positive charge on the molecule) before it can become part of the porphyrin ring.

HEMOGLOBIN CARRIER OXYGEN
IN BLOOD STREAM

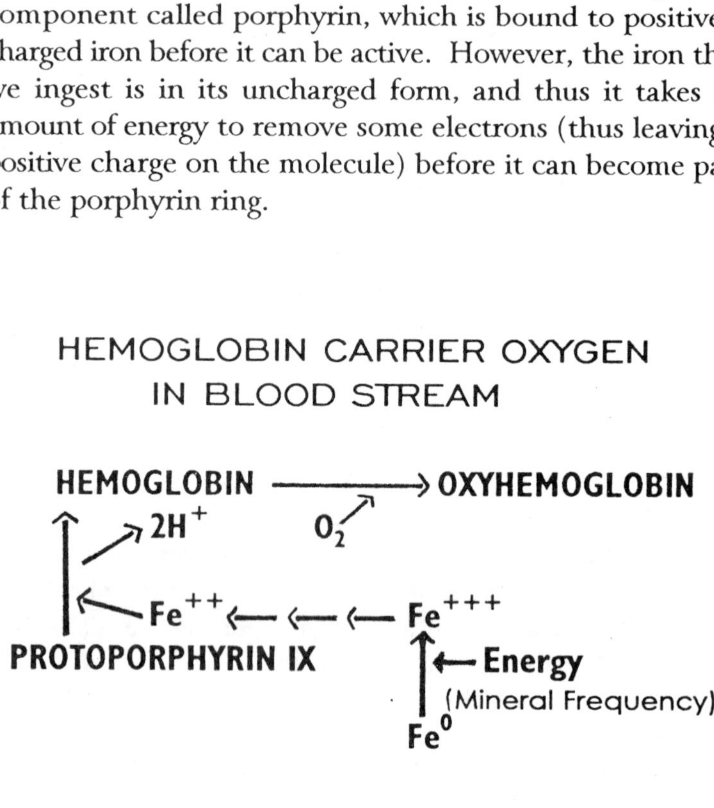

If the patient has nails that are very narrow and very light in color with a bottom that is dull yellow or dark blue, then this person has a skeletal problem. Narrow nails that are elongated with vertical ridges (whose significance will be discussed later) running along them, especially if they are dark-colored, tend to indicate respiratory disorders of a chronic nature (Fig. 1-b). If the nails are extremely narrow and elongated proportionally to the body, and a dark yellow or grey color, then it is even more indicative of the bone and skeletal problems mentioned above (Fig. 1-c).

A patient who has upside down triangularly-shaped nails that are light in color is prone to paralysis, especially if the nails are not blood-colored, or are a yellowish red color (Fig. 1-d). This patient may often feel numb and should be treated for paralysis.

A patient who has nails that are shaped like an upside-down triangle could also be experiencing symptoms of a stroke. This type of patient also runs a higher risk of acquiring paralysis. If the upside-down triangle is small, or red and large in the middle of the nail, then this patient is suffering from circulatory or bone marrow problems.

Slow growing nails with these symptoms may signify that the patient has cirrhosis, neuro-dermatitis, or a nail disease.

An extremely curved, clubbing nail is caused by lung disease, such as lung tumors or emphysema, where alveoli is not completely exchanging air (Fig. 1-e). This can also be detected if the nail appears to be completely opaque in color, and is especially indicative of emphysema. Here, hemoglobin has a low binding potential, causing insufficient oxygen exchange and too much carbon dioxide.

Short, wide, reddish nails (see Pic. 1-d, 2-a) signal cardiovascular problems including high blood pressure, atherosclerosis and the possibility of stroke or brain hemorrhage.

Curvature

Curvatures of the nail should be horizontally arched. If there happens to be no arch, or if the middle of the nail curves bidirectionally causing the nail to grow inward, then the patient may be suffering from emphysema, if the nail is raised in the middle and then curves downward, also called clubbing (Fig. 1-e). It could also signify that the patient has rheumatoid arthritis. Some nails may be concave with the tip going up. This may indicate anemia, if the nail is dipped inward and then curves upward (Fig. 1-f).

A patient who has clubbing fingernails and also has opaque nails definitely is suffering from a pulmonary heart disease such as serious emphysema, tuberculosis, congenital heart diseases, liver cirrhosis, or malignant tumors. If the opaque nails turn thick, hard and begin to lose its luster, then this person may be experiencing external trauma such as a fungus infection or several congenital diseases. Thick, yellow nails that grow at an extremely slow pace signify respiratory, lymphatic, or thyroid problems.

3

NAIL COLOR

Nail color can often be used to show a person's health, or give evidence of disorders the person maybe suffering. A healthy, energetic person should have slightly flexible, pink-colored nails that are shiny and strong. On the other hand, a person who suffers from malnutrition or anemia has nails that are very pale and shows no signs of the fast, healthy blood circulation that should be present. For instance, a patient who has just undergone surgery usually has no color in her nails. A person whose nails have changed from yellow to green to black has a chronic disease in her internal organs. For instance, a patient who is severely ill will have nails that are completely covered in a dark, near-black tint.

The following subheadings indicate what disorders correlate to each of the different fingernail colorings seen in patients.

White Nails

Nails that are usually white signify that the patient suffers from anemia. A person who has nails that are waxy in appearance in addition to having a white color to them may have other problems as well. This appearance, along with nails that are opaque, and are lacking in luster, may indicate that the patient suffers from ulcers, hemorrhaging, or hookworms.

Some patients may have a white color on part of their nails but not on the entire area of the nails. This condition can indicate other disorders. Nails that are white throughout most of the area except for the tips signify that the person may suffer from liver cirrhosis.

If the nails are not exactly white but are more of a cloudy, opaque color, then this should be indicative of a heart or lung problem. Further indication of this would be if the nails appear to be clubbing, in which the end of the nail is raised, then once past the flesh curves down on the fingertips.

Yellow Nails

Yellow nails may often signify liver, digestive problems, mainly due to jaundice caused by hepatitis or a chronic bleeding disease (Pic. 2-b). This may also be caused by other problems, such as:
1) hyperthyroidism, kidney problems, nail fungus, or an excess of Beta Carotene
2) water retention in the lymphatic system, especially possible if the nail has a slow growth-rate.
3) hair loss if the color of the nails are almost of a copper color (see Lily Hair Tonic in Appendix A)
4) melanoma, liver problems, or poor digestive functions if the tip of the nail is yellow instead of white. These people, who are normally smokers, tend to have taken an excessive

amount of tetracycline.

Red Nails

Redness of the nails can sometimes be attributed to the function of the circulatory system, but there are many different systems whose problems may result in the redness of all or parts of the nails.

If the colors of the nails are reversed, that is, switched so that the part of the nail over the lunula and matrix is red and the rest of the nail is actually white, then this patient has a circulation or heart problem and also may be prone to coughing, with other symptoms that include vomiting blood (Fig. 2-a). If the color of the nails appear to be completely red, then the patient may have heart disease, or lung disease (Fig. 2-b). If there are red spots underneath the nails, then the patient may be experiencing capillary vessel bleeding, high blood pressure, skin problems, or heart diseases.

If the circumference of the nails are covered with reddish bruises, then this patient may be suffering from a lupus infection or dermatitis. If the front of the nail is covered by a red band, then this signifies that the patient's gastrointestinal tract should be treated from inflammation. This condition may also signify that the patient is suffering from a heart valve problem. If the nail is dark red and does not form a triangle even with applied pressure, then the patient's organs may be experiencing inflammation.

If a patient notices that, when pressing down on the tip of the fingernails, that the blood still carries over, then this means that the artery valve isn't closing well and that there is an accumulation of old blood beyond the area. This symptom also signifies that the veins are not functioning properly and that the patient may be experiencing hyperthyroidism.

A patient may be suffering from carbon monoxide poisoning if the flesh beneath her nails, as well as her lips and cheeks are a bright cherry red color.

Purple Nails

Purple nails usually signify that the patient lacks oxygen and suffers from circulatory problems. This condition generally stems from either congenital, hereditary disorders, or from habitual problems such as lack of exercise and hence low oxygen saturation levels on a cellular level. The color will tend to be darker and ruddier than if the nails were to be diagnosed with a reddish color; these nails will look unhealthy as well, often lacking luster.

If the nails are purple and are covered with dots, then this patient may also be prone to suffering from cramps in various parts of the body, particularly in the extremities.

Green/Blue Nails

Green/blue nails suggest that the patient has an acute abdominal problem and often suffers from cold extremities. A patient with this coloring could also be experiencing food or drug poisoning. Nails that are of this color have also been associated with early stages of cancer.

Green Nails

Nails of this color often suggest irritation caused by cleansing agents or detergents. A patient with these symptoms could also be suffering from bacillus infections. Greenish or purplish colored nails could also signal a serious case of emphysema.

Blue Nails

Nails of this color are usually due to a lack of hemoglobin binding to oxygen, resulting in the bluish tint of venous blood, slow and deoxygenated. A patient with nails of this color often suffers from copper poisoning, or gas poisoning which can bind to hemoglobin competitively and make the oxygen-carriers dysfunctional.

Besides poisoning, a patient with this symptom could also suffer from rheumatoid arthritis or autoimmune diseases such as lupus. It would be beneficial to use other techniques to verify the condition.

If nails are a dark blue or reddish color, showing coagulated blood, then this may be due to prior strokes, high blood lipids, atherosclerosis, lower ability to keep blood thin, liver cirrhosis or hepatitis. Post symptoms of hepatitis, or kidneys having clogged capillaries, thrombosis or inflammation, or high platelet count. These types of people have higher chances of coronary heart disease and brain embolism.

Brown Nails

Nails have a tendency to turn a brown or dark brown color due to copper or arsenic poisoning. These nails may also have spotty indentations and could be due to a dry fungal infection. The cause of these dry fungal infections are not always clear, but they have to do with the general condition of the body.

Grey Nails

A patient with nails of this color could be experiencing arthritis or problems which show symptoms of edema. Grey nails have also been shown to be associated with malnutrition and post-operative effects on the body.

A grey color that spreads into the root area of the nail, where the matrix and lunulae are found, tends to signify that the patient has glaucoma.

Nails that are greyish-white usually indicate that the person has lung problems. A person with this symptom may also have emphysema or cardio-pulmonary disease (possible congenital or environmental diseases).

Black Nails

Black nails are often caused by trauma, or are signs of silver deposits. Bacteria infection will also cause the blackness in the nails. If the tip of the nail is black, then this suggests that the patient could be suffering from chronic kidney failure. A patient with this nail color may also be suffering from a lack of B12 vitamin and/or a lowered level of adreno-cortico steroids. Most importantly, if the thumbnails and toenails have black edges or black lines that vertically cover the nails, then the patient must be checked immediately by a physician, as many melanoma patients display this type of condition. If the nails are opaque, glassy, and blackish-red in color, then this person has a chronic kidney problem.

4

RIDGES, BUMPS AND OTHER MARKINGS ON THE NAILS

Ridges, bumps and white spots on the fingernail point to several potential problems in areas such as the adrenal glands, the liver, kidney, the endocrine hormones, etc., and can locate problems such as arthritis, parasites, and respiratory diseases. Unlike popular belief, these spots and ridges are not all caused by simple zinc or calcium deficiency, which is what most people tend to ascribe the appearance. Unfortunately, many of these patients who are prescribed zinc or calcium supplements for their condition see no improvement even after prolonged usage of the minerals. Zinc has been shown to be good for fertility, but white marks on the nail are a type of disorder that requires more comprehensive coverage of the excretory system as well.

Ridges and dips

A person who has vertical or horizontal ridges that are not very noticeable has no need to worry. They are perfectly normal. It is also commonly seen in patients over the age of forty. These ridges, especially if they are on the thumbs, can often be attributed to kidney problems (Fig.1-a, Pic.1-a). However, if the vertical or horizontal ridges are blatantly noticeable, then this patient may be suffering from an illness and the ridges are symptoms of the disease.

Vertical ridges that cover most of the fingernails refer to nerve or respiratory system problems (Fig.1a; Pic.1-b, 2-b). These ridges are commonly seen in old age, but this does not imply that they are a natural part of the aging process. Proper health care can prevent these ridges from forming. If the vertical ridges appear only on the thumbs then they refer to excretory system conditions. Ridges that are on only the four fingers except for the thumb are due to respiratory problems. An entire nail covered with vertical ridges could be caused by trauma sustained by the patient, either recently or as early as years past. If the ridges are very conspicuous, then the patient may be suffering from peripheral blockage, a particular yeast or fungus infection, or a hair follicle corneum.

Vertical indentations and black lines across the nails that appear in a youthful person may be nothing to worry over as the person develops. However, if these signs appear in a person after the age of 30, then one should be careful of possible problems. If only one or two of the nails appear to be in this condition, then this is not really cause to worry. However, if all of the nails are like this, then it could be indicative of Addison's disease, chronic adreno-cortico insufficiency. With this comes a poor appetite, vomiting, and also serious fatigue and weight loss. A patient with vertical lines across the faces of his nails could also suffer from Vitamin A deficiency or a chronic inflammation.

If the nails have vertical ridges that can be very easily split down the middle, this could be due to adrenal gland problems. For those that are under the age of forty, and in young people in general, vertical ridges definitely indicate problems in the bodily system. These types are usually chronically fatigued, nervous, and suffer neurasthenia. These young people also possibly suffer bronchitis, asthma, or laryngitis. In these people, ridges on the thumb signal those who have spleen and heart problems and may be depressed. Those on the index finger signal unhappiness in the patient, while middle finger ridges show nervousness and hyperactivity. Vertical ridges on the ring finger signal the possibility that the patient is heartbroken or suffering emotional trauma, while those on the pinky nail show long time stress and the overexertion of energy leading to liver and kidney damage.

Ridges in either direction may be caused by anemia, irregular kidney function, kidney failure, lupus, or be the effects of chemotherapy. Radiation therapy and excessive drug-use, both prescription and illicit, will affect kidney function and result in anomalies. Markings will show these to also be effects that come along with disorders that result in connective tissue cell differentiation and nutrient absorption deviations. If one is dieting, these markings will be caused by malnourishment.

Nails that become detached from the flesh of the fingers as they grow, or ridgy growth in nails, may both be caused by a fungal infection. More accurately, it is said to be caused by imperfect cell differentiation and poor capillary circulation, allowing fungus to invade and cause widespread infection.

Nails that are thin with high edges and a dip in the middle

(like a spoon) reveals a system that suffers from hemoglobin deficiency (Fig. 1-f) (Pic.2-a). A person with symptoms such as these may also be suffering from anemia or rheumatoid fever, or contain hookworms or syphilis. All of these symptoms also tend to portray hyperthyroidism.

If the nail has bumpy, raised dots, with an appearance similar to beads on a string,(see Pic.1-a) these are often due to arthritis or rheumatoid arthritis (Fig. 2-c). Nails that are covered with slight bumps and have an uneven face are usually due to psoriasis or eczema. Also, if the bumps grow without nails, then this patient may be suffering from congenital trauma or perpetual infections.

How do horizontal ridges appear? Horizontal ridges on the nails are typically due to poor blood circulation or poor growth and development, or in my opinion, a consequence of stress and sudden changes in diet. If the body is suffering from a condition or ailment that allows the nails to grow slower, then the body returns to normal and the nail growth rate speeds up again, this causes horizontal lines in the nail to appear, as the nail starts and stops growth.

Horizontal lines across the nails could also signify that the person either suffers from malnutrition, measles, or mumps (Fig. 2-d,e)(Pic. 2-c). If the nails are covered with numerous horizontal lines and with bumps like a washboard, then the patient may be suffering from a matrix/cuticle inflammation, or matrix damage. This may also signify that the patient suffers from some kind of pressure from a tumor or trauma.

Horizontal white lines are most commonly caused by chronic kidney problems (Pic. 2-d). This condition is particularly noticeable if the patient has more than one horizontal white line with a fuzzy appearance. However, horizontal white lines can be the result of many other things, such as:
1) arsenic or lead poisoning, and/or
2) Hutchinson's disease.

A patient who has deep horizontal dips is likely to have suffered from one of two possibilities if it is not due to a major illness or external damage on the hand (Fig. 2-d,e). If these horizontal dips are very shallow but continuous over the nail, they signify that the patient either lacks certain essential nutrients, which are necessary to good health and healthy nails, or has poor circulation and heart disease, in which the nail will have usually one very deep dip. However, stress is also a factor that can cause many shallow horizontal lines. The ages of these horizontal dips can be determined by their depth and nail-coverage (Pic.1-c). One can estimate approximately when the problem happened by measuring the distance of the dip from the matrix, or bottom of the nail. For adults, it usually takes six months to grow the entire nail. In Fig.2-e, you can see that, based on the location of the dips, the problem took place about 2-3 months ago.

Spots and Markings

White spots that appear on the nails of men, women, and children may have to do with kidney and hormonal imbalances (Pic. 3-a). Zinc and calcium deficiencies are also possible, as most holistic doctors feel, but this is not necessarily all that is the case. In children and adolescents, this may be due to developmental changes or hormonal changes that occur in the normal growth stages (which is also seen in menopause, another natural phase.) This changing can also cause air bubbles to form underneath the nails, which should not cause alarm.

Other reasons for white spots are excessive chemical or drug use which would cause the kidneys to be overworked to try to cleanse the system. These patients will need extreme detoxifying and should take Asparagus Extract, Chi Energy, and use mineral infrared treatment on the kidney area of the lower back to help aid filtration and kidney function. Another indication of poor kidney function is the presence of fuzzy white strips running horizontally across the nail (Pic.2-a), signaling the chance of protein and excess nitrogen in the urine. (Another way to discuss the presence of protein in the urine will be discussed in part III.) In these cases, Asparagus Extract has been shown to be very helpful, as can be expressed by a doctor in Arkansas who used it on a patient already needing dialysis. Within three days, the patient's kidney had improved so remarkably that he was able to urinate on his own once again.

Genital infections such as chlamydia and syphilis can also cause white spots. In men who are in their late 30's or 40's, spots may mean prostate problems or forthcoming impotence. (Studies show that 1 out of every 8 American men are impotent.) Prostate problems can also be signaled if the patient must go to the bathroom over once per night under the age of 55. In this case, mineral infrared therapy is good for helping the disorder, as well as other herbs which treat the prostate.

Nails that are covered with grey dots signify that this patient suffers from dry nail fungus, a condition known as tinea which is also related to hair loss, alopecia, and other autoimmune diseases. A person with nail fungus should consult a specialist and attain treatment for the condition before it worsens. One way to tell whether or not the fungal infection has spread throughout the body is to press the associated meridian points and test for sensitivity: either on the insides of the thighs halfway between the hip and the knee, or in the notch where the collarbone meets the shoulder blade. If one feels a sharp pain, this means that she has a low immunity and a systemic candida infection. At this point, it would be very beneficial to take Asparagus Extract and/or Maitake (See Appendix A).

If one has fuzzy looking white splotches, like little elliptical patterns, this signals the possibility of a condition such as incontinence, any genital or uterine infection, or sexually transmitted diseases that carries symptoms such as white discharge. This may also signal vaginitis, in which case Happy Skin Tonic may be very good for washing and douching (See Appendix A).

If the middle fingernail has red spots on it, this could be due to a heart problem (Fig.2-f). This problem is seen in many patients, and is one that doctors should be especially aware of. If this condition is seen, then other symptoms of the same disorder should be checked to confirm the suspicion. If nail has dark line which moves when nail grows, it is internal bleeding or ulcers (Fig. 3-a). If spotch shows on the nail, and not move with nail growth, it could be cancer.

5

Lunulae

The first and most important factor when diagnosing fingernails is to look at the lunulae on the nails, the small white half-moons at the bottom of the nail. These lunulae represent the cellular oxygen levels in the patient, and can tell whether or not there is proper oxygen saturation intra cellularly. Each person should be able to see eight (8) lunulae on their fingernails, 4 on each hand. These lunulae should also be of a certain length; they should not be too large or too small. Absence of one of more lunulae, or smaller lunulae than normal, signal a deficiency in cellular oxygen levels. This type of deficiency leads to symptoms such as cold hands, cold feet, and sometimes a general numbness in certain parts of the body. The patient feels weak and fatigued, with many cases of memory loss. In this bodily condition, there are greater associated cases of candidas infection and cancer. Poor circulation could be caused by circulatory blockage, which may be due to the presence of toxic heavy metals or the accumulation of triglycerides and other lipids in the system.

As I mentioned before, a healthy person should have eight lunulae, small moon-like white areas at the bottom of the nail. The existence of lunulae means that that particular area of tissue is saturated with oxygen. Each lunulae is led by meridian lines to the areas of the body they represent. If the fingernail has no lunulae, it signifies a lack of oxygen saturation in cells, which must not be confused with shallowness of breath or any other voluntary process. Thus, any administration of such substances as ozone and hydrogen peroxide will not help the oxygen situation. If your tissues are not completely saturated with oxygen, it is due to some sort of circulatory or lymphatic system blockage and needs to be cleared as soon as possible to prevent further damage.

Lunulae also represent a person's Chi (or Qi) energy, a term the Chinese use to mean a form of bodily energy, referring specifically to a person's spirit and inner strength. Lunulae should appear on all fingers but the pinkies. The size of the lunulae on the thumb should be much larger in area than that on any other finger. The Lunulae should, beginning with the thumb and ending with the ring finger, decrease in size and should take up no more than 1/4 the size of the nail. Size of the lunula is due to lung function varieties. This has to do with oxygen uptake and the cell's own oxidation potentials and aging potential. Hormone functions are also lower with smaller lunulae.

Many people feel that oxygen therapy or ozone therapy is beneficial to their health. This is true only in the case that the person's circulation is good. However, if there are large lunulae on every fingernail (including the pinky nail, where there should not be a lunulus,) and especially if there is also a noticeable reddish strawberry-like area or narrow, pointy tip at the front of the tongue, then these patients have a high chance of heart disease and other heart conditions. These people are hyperexcitable and generally have a ruddy complexion. Stroke is also possible if the lunulae are oversized and quite large. A person has a greater chance of having a stroke if the lunulae on one hand are markedly smaller than those on the other. This, though common in people who use one hand much more than the other (i.e. writers, pitchers, etc.) can also indicate the possibility that one side of the body has a circulation blockage that does not affect the other side. If the problem worsens, risk of a stroke is greatly increased, and is more likely to occur on the side of the blockage. If all the lunulae are extremely large, seemingly reaching the tip of the nail to the point where there is but a little bit of red left, this could be indicative of liver cirrhosis.

If there are less than 8 lunulae on all the fingernails, then there is a problem with poor circulation. A patient who is lacking lunulae on between 3 and 7 fingernails often has symptoms of fatigue and has low energy, is weak-spirited. This condition also show poor circulation, cold hands and feet, numbness, and memory loss. A patient who has 2 large lunulae on the pinkies has a very over-worked heart and is more prone to suffer from high blood pressure and heart disease than a healthy person. A person who has no lunulae at all often suffers from anemia, depression, and low blood pressure.

Finally, a thyroid problem can be seen if a person's lunulae has a shoot-like growth sprouting from its border (Fig.3-b) This is quite accurate and can be seen in other thyroid problem indications.

6

DIAGNOSIS BY SYSTEM

Fingernail diagnosis is grouped by system and problem below, so that one can confirm the correct general conditions upon checking the following categories after examination:

Cardiovascular problems:

Short, wide, reddish nails signal cardiovascular problems including high blood pressure, atherosclerosis and the possibility of stroke or brain hemorrhage.

If the tops of the nails are wide while the bottoms of the nails are much narrower, this could be indicative of the possibility of stroke and other cardiovascular problems. Stroke is also possible if the lunulae are oversized and quite large.

If there are less than 8 lunulae on all the fingernails, then there is a problem with poor circulation. Patients exhibiting problems of this sort should take Vein Lite to increase blood circulation and repair the lack of oxygen intracellularly.

Respiratory problems:

If the nails have a rolled appearance, with tips that curl upwards and a surface that resembles rough glass in its opacity and texture, then this is indicative of respiratory problems such as emphysema.

If the colors of the different parts of the nails are reversed, with the lunulae being reddish while the rest of the nail is whitish, then the patient may have respiratory problems such as bronchitis.

Greenish or purplish colored nails signal a serious case of emphysema along with various other respiratory disorders. Ridges along the nails also signal respiratory problems, and perhaps are indicative of kidney problems as well.

Digestive problems:

If the nail is flattened instead of being slightly curved in appearance, then this signals digestive problems such as chronic gastritis.

If the nail is blackish or yellowish in tone, then the patient may have a digestive problem (Fig. 3-c)(Pic.2-b). This problem may not necessarily be simply a fungal infection.

If the middle nail has a red elongated or circular spot in the upper corner, then this is possibly indicative of chronic gastritis (Fig. 2-f). If the ring finger on the right hand has a black circular or oval spot in the middle of the nail, then this is indicative of liver problems, and even liver cancer. If there are ridges that appear on the fingernails, this may also be indicative of a liver problem.

Kidney and Sex Hormone problems:

If the nails show two horizontal white lines going across the entire nail, then this is indicative of chronic kidney problems or low blood protein (Pic. 2-c).

Ridges, which can sometimes be blackish or colored, and white spots on the fingernail indicate kidney problems and hormonal problems.

If the nails are a greenish color, then if the patient is pregnant, the child may have serious problems, and perhaps be stillborn.

If the nails are quite short naturally, but the color still normal, then the patient may be infertile.

Arthritis:

If there are vertical ridges on the nail and the nail is bumpy, causing a beaded-string effect on the texture of the nail surface, then the patient may have rheumatoid arthritis or arthritis.

If the nail resembles an upside down triangle, then this is indicative of rheumatoid arthritis. Many of these bone and joint conditions, including this one and others including osteoporosis, can be treated with mineral infrared therapy to increase adrenal gland activity, which in turn produces hormones which work toward healthier bones.

Eye problems:

If the thumbnails have grey-colored markers and a wave-like appearance on the left sides, then this is indicative of glaucoma in the patient.

Parasites:

If then nail is shaped like a spoon, that is, has concave surface instead of a convex one, then the possibility of the patient having anemia or parasites such as tapeworms, is quite likely.

Nails that are whitish, dull in luster, and waxy-looking are quite possibly due to the presence of tapeworms in the system or other parasites.

Bone problems:

Nails that are atrophied, shriveled, and thin, are indicative of spinal problems in the patient such as osteoporosis.

Blood problems:

This is similar to the symptoms and descriptions seen in parasitic invasions, in which the nail has vertical ridges and is shaped like a spoon that is concave instead of convex, is easily torn or split, and which signals an bodily mineral deficiency (Pic.2-b), and anemic conditions.

If the nail is yellow and lacking in the color of blood, then the patient has chronic internal bleeding.

This description is similar to that of certain respiratory problems, in that the colors of the different parts of the nails are reversed, except that the patient has the added symptom of vomiting blood.

Nervous System disorders:

If the patient's nails show no lunulae at all, then the patient may have neurasthenia, or depression, experiencing weakness and fatigue; patient may be prone to cancer.

If the thumbnail has red or purple stripes on the right side, then the patient the patient may be prone to migraines.

If the thumb is all or partially grey in color and opaque, then the patient's symptoms may include frequent dizziness and fainting.

Autoimmune Diseases:

If the root or matrix area of the nails are redbluish-colored and rough, the center of the nail is raised, the tip is curved upward, then the patient may have an autoimmune disease (Fig. 3-d) such as lupus, rheumatoid arthritis, psoriasis, eczema, etc. This description is similar to the appearance in the case of respiratory disorders, where the nail is opaque, grey, and curling over onto itself while raised in the middle. This type of description is usually associated to patients with severe emphysema, or cancer.

Lymphatic System problems:

If the nail is slow-growing, thick, and hard, with a curved

surface area and dull luster, this is indicative of a problem in the lymphatic system.

If the nail is greenish, then the body is poisoned and the possibility of cancer is great.

Bone Marrow disorders:

If the nails are oval shaped instead of the normal shape, then this is significant of bone marrow dysfunction.

Thyroid disorders:

If the patient has the description similar to that of parasites in that the nail has a spoon-like shape that is concave rather than convex, it could also signal thyroid imbalance.

If the fingernails are brittle and easily broken, this is indicative of thyroid problems (Fig. 3-e). Also, shoot-like growths from the lunulae also signal this problem (Fig. 3-b).

Adrenal Gland disorders:

If the patient's fingernails have ridges and are easily split and torn, then this could signal some problem in the adrenal gland (Fig. 3-f, Pic.2-b).

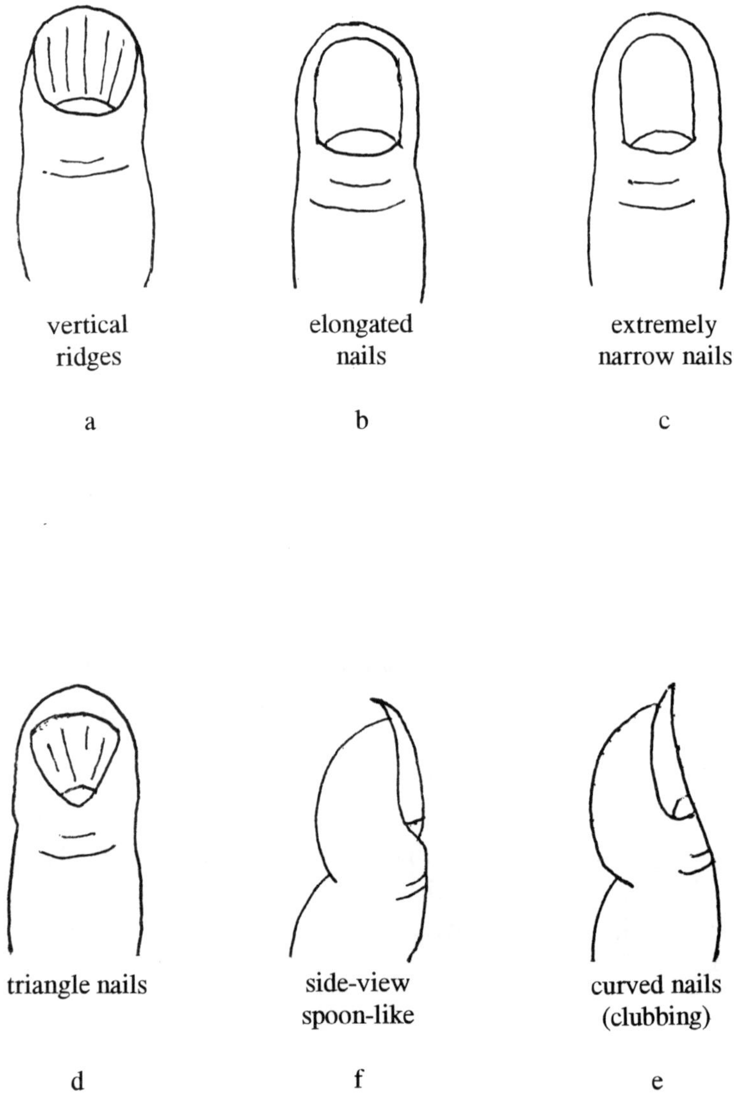
vertical ridges
a
elongated nails
b
extremely narrow nails
c
triangle nails
d
side-view spoon-like
f
curved nails (clubbing)
e

Fig 1

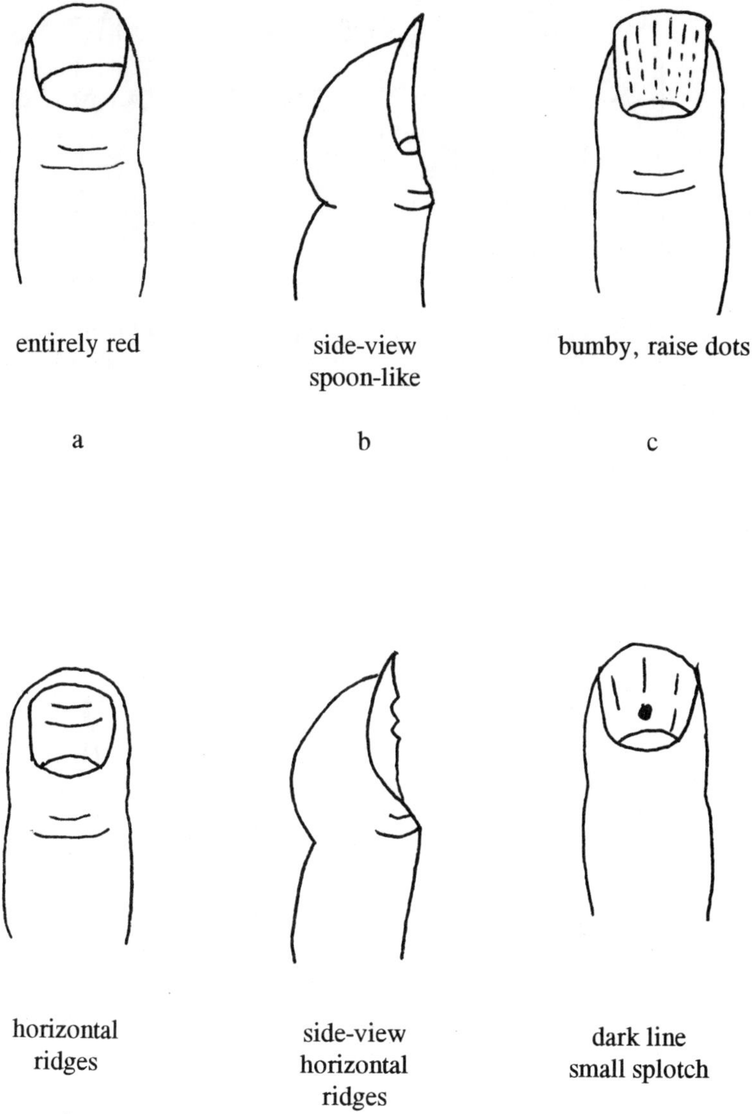
entirely red
a
side-view
spoon-like
b
bumby, raise dots
c
horizontal
ridges
d
side-view
horizontal
ridges
e
dark line
small splotch
f

Fig 2

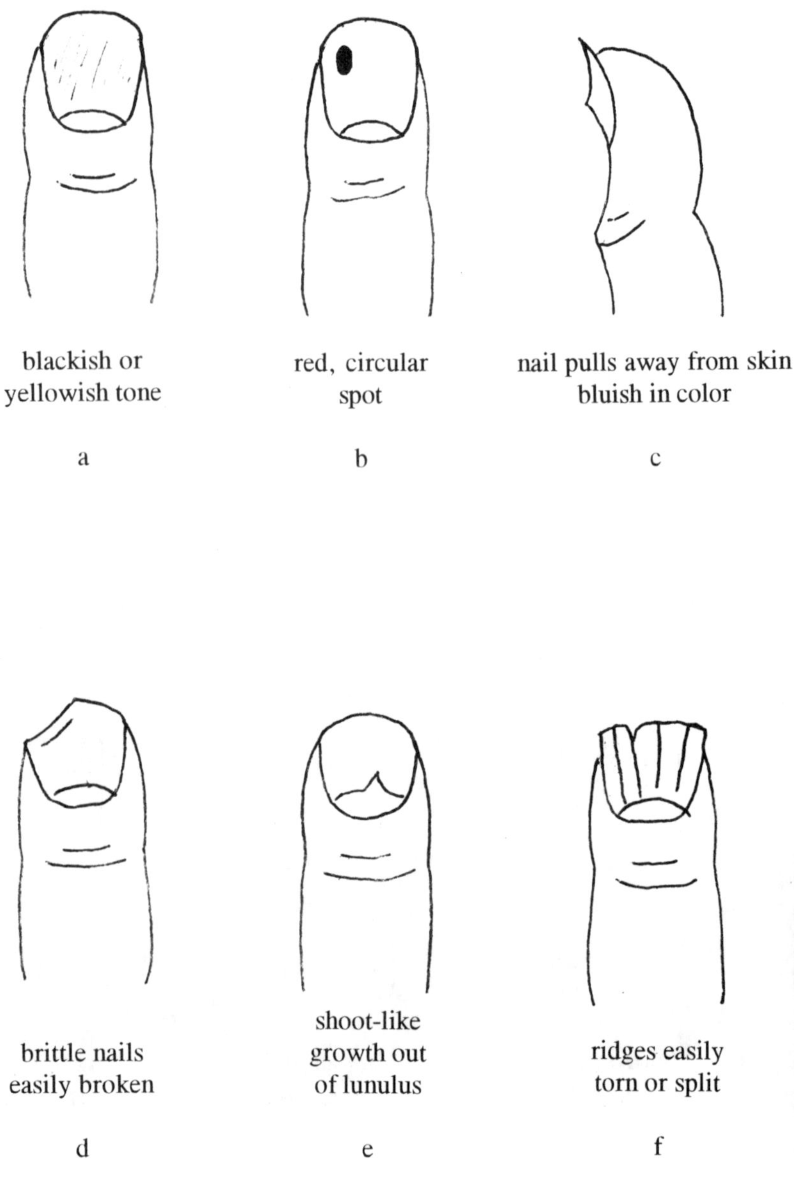
blackish or
yellowish tone
a
red, circular
spot
b
nail pulls away from skin
bluish in color
c
brittle nails
easily broken
d
shoot-like
growth out
of lunulus
e
ridges easily
torn or split
f

Fig 3

Part II

Tongue Diagnosis

7

Overview of the Tongue Diagnosis

The method of tongue diagnosis can be described as one of Chinese and Indian Ayurvedic techniques toward long term disease prevention and good health. The Chinese have used it for thousands of years, and as recently as the 19th century, Western doctors also looked at patients' tongues during examinations, though in a different manner in that it was used as a much more specific medical marker. The Western method of checking the tongue has since phased out, but it is actually a very important part of a general exam that should be reinstated in a modified form, so that both Western and Eastern thought can be incorporated to arrive at an exciting and remarkably accurate medium by coordinating the symptoms to the problems.

Generally, the appearance of the tongue can give valuable information on organ function, and is done by looking at various components of it. The tongue should be examined everyday before or after brushing the teeth to look for problems. Many meridian lines run along the tongue, and thus the tongue is an important location of bodily function. When the body is not functioning correctly, it is reflected on the tongue. For instance, one often notices that during sickness, the tongue will appear duller and perhaps even a different color and texture than when one is healthy. Similarly, the tongue may appear bloated when the body is experiencing edema elsewhere or disorders which would cause water retention.

The tongue is the most visible internal member of the body. The topmost layer of epithelial tissue is constantly growing and replacing old tissue with new. The entire layer takes only 2-3 days to become fully replaced, and the regeneration of tissue is fast enough to be compared with that of the small intestines. Since this growth is so fast, the cells' metabolism must also be high, so any malnutrition or ailment in the body can be quickly seen on the tongue. The lack of necessary nutrients such as the vitamin B group, vitamin C, iron, and zinc all cause oxidation of cells and thus a change in the cells themselves. Taste cells also become atrophied as malnourishment progresses. Oftentimes, these changes are so immediate that they can be detected and followed before any other changes in the body occur.

Another reason that the tongue is so indicative of the body's condition is the fact that the tongue contains a lot of blood vessels and thus reflects the condition of the blood in the body. If the constituents of the blood change even slightly, then this change will show on the tongue very clearly, resulting in a color change that is noticeable almost immediately.

We shall begin by clarifying the exact way in which to examine one's tongue. To begin, the patient should have a clean mouth that has been brushed recently but preferably not immediately prior to the examination. This way the tongue will not bear any temporary marks or color changes to the palette which may affect its normal appearance. The patient should not have eaten anything immediately prior to the examination as well, as this can also affect both the color and the texture of the tongue, depending on the consistency and the color of food eaten. The tongue should be extended out of the mouth evenly, with the tip pointed downwards, and a flat palette. The patient must be careful so as not to stretch the tongue so far that the blood flow is affected. The general quality of the tongue should be noted first and foremost: its color, thickness and whether or not there is a coating present. If there is a coating, observation may be made regarding whether or not the coating extends over the entire tongue, or whether it is patchy, indicating a condition known as a geographical tongue, or sparsely located throughout. Next the details of the tongue must be examined, noting symptoms of disorder such as bleeding, bruised spots, or lesions. The movements and facultative ability of the tongue must be noted as well.

By looking at the vitality of the tongue, the body color, shape, coating, and moisture level, one can determine the condition of the patient as it relates to the 5 systems. The tongue has been found to be a quite consistent marker in examining a person's health, and can be used to follow a patient's health improvement or decline. The tongue body color is generally used to detect chronic conditions while the quality of the coating of the tongue is used to detect acute conditions.

Vitality of the tongue

What is the inherent quality of the tongue? Is it generally healthy in spirit, or does it lag and appear tired and withered? Look especially at the root, or the very back, of the tongue(Pic.4-a). The movements of the tongue are also indicative of this kind of vitality, which is closely connected to brain coordination and motor function. If one is able to move the tongue back and forth, side-to-side, with full mobility, then this reflects astute motor function and good coordination functions of the brain. Any deviation from the proper ability to move the tongue signals deficiencies in coordination and brain function.

Body color

This is a very important component of the tongue analysis. This aspect of the tongue reflects what is known by the Chinese as the "Heat" of the system as opposed to the "Cold" characteristics in a person. The darker red the tongue is, the more Heat is associated to the condition. The paler the tongue appears, the more Cold is associated. Heat is often associated more with patients who have heart diseases or heart trouble of the sort, while Cold is often associated more with cancer patients and people with poor circulation. You can sometimes easily tell if a person is "hot" if they appear to have a generally ruddy complexion, which is sometimes seen as redness throughout the body as well. These people will also tend to be "hotter" in terms of temper and disposition as well, having more emotional flare-ups than the colder types. Cold types, on the other hand, generally are seen as having sallow, pale complexions and are much more inactive than those that are considered in Chinese medicine to be hot. Simply put, cold type people just feel and emanate the typically "colder" characteristics, while hot type people are just plain "hotter," in most senses of the word. Hot and cold descriptions in Chinese medicine have a lot to do with the circulation of the patient.

In a healthy individual, the tongue should have a solid, fleshy pink color. If the tongue is paler or white instead, then there is poor circulation and the person may even be anemic. On the other hand, if the tongue is dark in color, with a red or even purple flare, then this may signal circulation blockages due to poisons in the system, or heavy metals in the body which must be removed.

Body shape

Looking at the tongue body's shape entails examining the shape as well as the features of the tongue including the texture and markings on the tongue.

By looking at the ridges, spots, and/or bumps that may be on the tongue, one can distinguish which part of the body is troubled. (See Chart B) Generally, markings or deformities on the tip of the tongue point to the heart area, while those on the front sides show lung-related problems, and those in the center of the tongue are related to gastro-intestinal and spleen problems. The edges along the very back of the tongue direct to gall bladder and liver functions. There are kidney, urine bladder, or sex hormone-related problems if there is any abnormality on the root of the tongue. The underside of the tongue can signal circulation problems as well as liver problems, one of which could be the failure of the liver to properly detoxify the heavy-metals from the system.

TONGUE Diagnosis

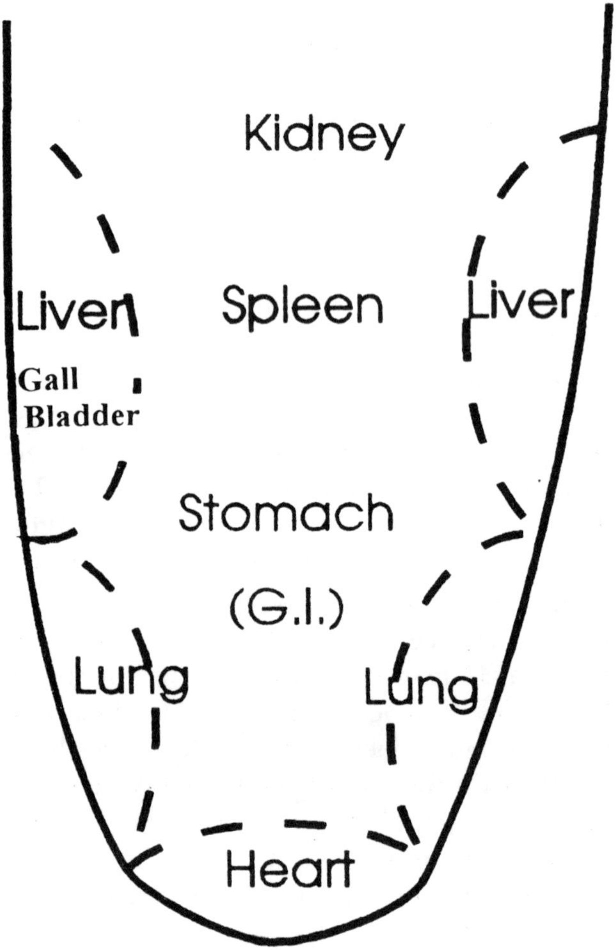

Chart B

Similarly, cracks in the tongue body will correlate to different systems of the body depending on their location, and the depth of such cracks signifies the severity of the condition. Cracks that are deeper than 2 mm are considered to be associated with very severe problems, while cracks that are less than 2 mm deep tend to have to do with more acute situations that are not are dire.

Perhaps the most important part to examining the shape of the tongue is noting the presence of teethmarks on the tongue, ridges along the side of the tongue which can point to spleen and other problems.

Tongue Coating

Tongue coating reflects the influential levels of Hot and Cold in the body, as well as the stage of the condition afflicting the patient. Healthy people should have a thin, whitish coating on the tongue that spreads over the entire palette. No coating on the tongue at all would signal a liver or kidney problem. Generally, the thicker the coating, the more extreme the situation. If the root has a coating but there are abnormalities elsewhere, the condition is usually acute. If there is not root coating, the condition is very serious, and if there is partial coating, or coating on one side only, then the condition is at an intermediate stage. If the abnormal coating is only at the tip of the tongue, then it is a mild problem. Generally, one should also be aware of the color of the tongue body itself, since tongue body color signals a more severe condition than that of the tongue coating. In other words, if the person has an abnormal tongue body color.

A healthy coating should consist of a thin whitish layer starting at the root of the tongue and thinning out as it approaches the tip. A thick coating all over the tongue signals respiratory problems; the thicker and more mucosy the coating is, the more extreme the conditions. A yellowish coating signals digestive problems, while a dark brownish/ greenish coating points to a liver problem. A purely dark green coating usually signals the accumulation of heavy metals such as francium oxide, which affects coenzyme A activity and sulfur amino acids. If the coating becomes bluish, then it is indicative of copper poisoning from pesticides or from the environment. Blackish coatings that cannot be easily scraped off are indicative of very serious liver and kidney problems. White coatings are usually indicative of respiratory problems or lung infections such as pneumonia.

Tongue Moisture

This provides information of the hydration of the body and the body's fluids. Normal tongues should only be slightly moist. Dryness indicates insufficiency of fluids (Pic. 3-b, which also indicates stomach problems), while wetness is indicative of accumulation of fluids, which are spleen/pancreas problems affecting the kidneys, showing teethmarks (Pic. 3-c). Smoking often produces a dry tongue, and this habit also tends to cause a general yellowish appearance of the tongue.

After checking the rest of the tongue, it is important to look at the frenula, the piece of tissue that connects the upper lip to the upper gums. If this piece of tissue has cyst-like growths on it, it signals digestive tract problems. If the growth is on the upper part of the frenula, this signals problems with the upper digestive pathway, such as the small intestine (Pic. 3-d). Growths on the lower frenula signal problems further along the digestive tract, such as in the large intestine and colon (see Pics. 4-b). This is caused by the fact that the liver may produce too much bile during digestion, which will accumulate in the intestines and become small secondary bile salts which is carcinogous, causing intestinal inflammation and ulcers. Cymosi Fibre-Cleanse can remove the bile salts (see Appendix A).

Lastly, but in no way of least importance, is the need to check the underside of the tongue, which can reveal much about the presence of toxins such as heavy metals in the body, seen as protruding and/or varicose veins on the bottom of the tongue (Pic. 4-c), because of too much carbon dioxide in the blood. Black veins also indicate acidity of the blood, which allows easy invasion of illnesses. Black or red spots on the bottom of the tongue are due to poisons and heavy metal accumulation (Pic.4-c,d).

8

Vitality and Movement of the Tongue

The general condition of the tongue is the first thing that should be observed when doing this type of examination. Vitality and quality of tongue tissue must be observed first and foremost to see if any problems can be immediately noticed. A healthy tongue is firm and fits proportionately into the bottom of the mouth. It should make movements with fluidity and strength, and show a firm capability to facilitate speech and any other movement. If the tongue is too soft and contains no vitality at all then the patient suffers from a secretory problem. The patient is lacking blood, fluid, or Chi (also called Qi, the Chinese term for overall bodily energy or strength). If the patient suffers from a lack of energy and fluid, then his meridians are not balanced. The softness of the tongue can related to any of the below causes: 1) saliva glands may not be producing enough saliva, 2) the nervous system may be experiencing problems, and 3) tongue muscles may be lacking in strength.

If the tongue is very stiff then the person's nerve transmissions are blocked and are thus unable to function properly. This type of person tends to be rather unstable and is easily annoyed. The stiffness of the tongue may be related to Type B meningitis, or if it is a high fever, then it may be related to liver coma or stroke. Patients with these symptoms must be treated right away.

If the tongue deviates from side to side then the patient

may be suffering from a cerebellum blood vessel stroke, hemorrhaging, tongue or facial nerves damage, or paralysis (Bell's Palsy). If the brain, facial, or liver problems are too strong, damage to the nervous system will be detrimental. Deviation of the tongue from side to side involuntarily is a pre-stroke symptom, and should be examined by a physician for preventative measures immediately.

If the tongue perpetually trembles involuntarily in shivering gestures, then the patient is lacking tongue energy, Chi, and blood and has a poor immune-system. The patients who suffer from tongue trembling have a hyperactive thyroid function and nerve damage. Old age can affect the nerves in the facial organs as well as the eyes, ears, nose, and mouth. Other causes of tongue trembling include poisoning by heavy metals such as mercury, manganese, barium, and chloride. Many heavy metals are found in the air we breathe, and are especially concentrated in gasoline, lead being the most obvious of these. Lead will cause headaches and insomnia, sweatiness and irregular periods as well. Mercury, also usually obtained through the air, can cause moodiness and gum problems with much saliva, and trembling in other parts of the body as well, including the fingers, eye, and legs. Many of the other heavy metals will cause such symptoms as hardening of the tongue, memory loss, and numbness.

Numbness of the tongue can be caused by methanol poisoning (which also leads to blindness) and/or thallium in the body, in the form of an acetate or sulfur derivative. These poisons will also cause peripheral bodily nerve irritation, loss of body hair and white nails.

If the patient's tongue is shriveled, then his basic tongue movement has been deterred. This type of patient usually suffers from acute myocardial infection. An infection of this kind often causes coma of certain kinds of brain diseases. If the patient has no saliva at all, then his condition is very dangerous.

If the tongue appears limp then the patient is lacking energy. A patient with this type of symptom is easily annoyed and is there is also a high occurrence of mental retardation among sufferers of this type. A patient with this condition may be suffering from toxemia, septicemia, or a low thyroid gland output and function. The results of these conditions may be enlarged extremities or poor refractive ability.

If the tongue is heavy because the veins on the underside protrude too much, the patient may be suffering from poor heart and stomach functions, as well as heavy metal poisoning (Pic. 4-b). The pH of the blood in these patients is quite acidic, thus allowing for easy infection of the bodily systems. Also, if the underside of the tongue reveals noticeable venous branching, this shows the likelihood of liver problems.

If the tongue moves slowly and appears to be curled under, then the patient has trouble talking. This is also known as cerebral vessel accident caused after-effects or meningitis. If the tongue cannot move in all directions quickly and coordinately, brain function is definitely lacking. People who have had a stroke may experience this type of inability to control the tongue movements as precisely as they once had, and may have less control over tongue.

9

Tongue Color

Distribution

It is important, when performing a tongue analysis, to be sure to check the tongue color, and the location thereof, as one of the main component of the method. The location and distribution of this color and texture has much to do with the situation of the person's health. Generally speaking, there are locations of back, front, left and right textured palettes. If the palette of the tongue spreads into the front area, it means that the disease is not too deep in the bodily system. If in the back, it is an inner organ disease due to phlegm, and poor digestive system. If it is only on the left side, (looking in), the organ is clogged. If the film is only on the right side, then the disease is throughout the body. So if the entire tongue is very, very thick there is lots of phlegm, then one will be able to confirm that the internal organs have problems also. If the tongue is thicker in the middle, that is normal. If it is only in the center, and nowhere else, these types have kidney and spleen problems.

Tongue Tip

If the tip of the tongue is dark or reddish, this indicates that the heart is of the "hot" characteristic. Other possible causes of this condition could be worrying too much, nervousness, hyperthyroid activity, acute appendicitis, or the occasional symptoms of PMS.

If the person is not diseased, and has a spotted tip, this is due to insomnia, or from eating tart or spicy food. If spots extend over the entire tongue, it signifies a female hormonal imbalance possibly due to puberty.

Clinically, if patients show an extreme case of these descriptions, this is likely to be due to hyperthyroid activity, measles, scarlet fever, or a possibility of any number of infectious external diseases which necessitates immediate physician's examination. Extreme cases may also signify infection about the thoracic membrane, bronchitis or any other upper respiratory infection, or neurasthenia.

Different Tongue Colors

Different overall tongue palette colors have been shown to be associated to different problems. The following is an outline of the symptoms and diseases that are associated with each of the different tongue palette colors:

If the tongue is YELLOW

Yellowness of the tongue signifies a problem in the stomach and spleen. Patients with yellow tongues generally have poor digestive system functions, so the stomach contains a lot of carbon dioxide from anaerobic fermentation. If the patient has recently eaten a lot of food with sulfur in it, after digestion, hydrogen sulfide will be exposed in the tongue, thus causing a yellowish tint. This in general is no need for worry. The worst case is if the palette becomes thicker-looking, signaling that the lymphocyte levels have increased, due to the presence of an array of possible infections and disease. If the liver and gall bladder are problematic, it will also show up as a green yellow or black yellow color, with abdominal bloating and pain upon pressure; nausea and constipation will also be prevalent in patients of this type.

Yellow, sticky-looking palette:
People with yellow palettes generally have bad breath and have more insensitive than normal taste buds. If extreme, there may be cracks in the tongue due to high temperatures in the body and the heat resulting from cell metabolism. This leads to fast production of epithelial cells, also quickly sloughing off old cells, causing cracks. There are some variegated symptoms of a yellow tongue:

Light yellow, moist-looking palette:
These patients are often thirsty, always warm, and sometimes experience light coughing. People with this color tongue often also experience the discomfort of a bloated abdomen and chest area.

Yellow, sticky-looking palette:
Patients will feel pain upon pressing the abdomen. They will have dry mouths but may not necessarily feel thirsty.

Yellow, dry-looking palette:
These patients like cold drinks. Their bodies are generally warm and sweaty. People with this color palette have a congested upper body.

Yellow, slimy-looking palette:
Patients will feel dry but not thirsty. People of this type will feel that their bodies are warm, faces red, chests congested.

If the tongue is GREY

This signifies that the patient's condition is far beyond that of a yellow-colored palette thus turning gray, signaling the advanced stages of a disease. These people are of yin power and have long lasting colds, weakened livers and spleens. In more extreme cases, there may be spikes and cracks on tongue, or the color may turn black. Infection by fungus: yeast or Candida will cause hydrogen sulfide production causing yellow and finally a gray color. These people have been shown to have a tendency to overuse broad spectrum antibiotics, causing resistance.

Gray, sticky-looking palette:
These patients suffer from a lot of chest congestion, and may feel waves of heat pass over them. They are very nauseous, quite thirsty and drink a lot of water; though they may sweat a lot, they generally do not urinate a lot. These problems are usually stemming from the lungs and respiratory system.

Gray, slimy-looking palette:
These patients have bloated abdomens, a sallow complexion, and are generally fatigued. They generally do not have a lot of urine, and experience cold shudders, especially in the area of the extremities.

Grayish-yellow colored palette:

Patients will feel their chest congested and nauseous but not vomitous. They are also easily annoyed, and may have dark, dense urine and a dry mouth but not be overly thirsty; diuretic action is strong.

Grayish-black tongue:
Patients will be feverish and experience headaches; the heart, lung, spleen and stomach are all in bad condition. Those with this color tongue also tend to be irritable, hyperactive and always thirsty. They also tend to have a reddish complexion and dry mouth, and often also a swollen throat.

If the tongue is WHITE

People with whitish tongues, and this must not be confused with having a whitish coating, (see chapter on Tongue Coating,) have this lack of color due to low or weak blood supply, which may caused by anemia or malnourishment. This could also be caused by parasites, kidney renalitis, edema, hemorrhaging, retarded adrenal cortex function, or unbalanced hormones. Protein catabolism function is low in this type and capillary circulation is poor as well.

If the tongue is RED

The normal color of a healthy tongue is light red, signaling good circulation and a healthy blood supply. However, if one has a blood red tongue, then most likely this abnormality stems from the fact that the person is a hot type character. If the tongue tip is more red than the rest of the tongue, this may be caused by a heart problem. If the sides of the tongue are reddest, this signifies a liver and gall bladder problem. If the whole tongue is red, and if there is no palette or the patient experiences dry mouth, then it is a stomach problem.

Redness in the tongue may also be due to bacteria which could have infected the blood and caused an acute infectious disease, pus in the blood or organs, a hyperthyroid condition, hypertension, diabetes, tuberculosis, hypermetabolism, or post-operative dehydration. Bodily nutrition is confused and dehydration is rapid, so blood cohesiveness is higher, showing up on the tongue as possible spikes or lesions, or blood spots. The tongue could have an upside down T-shaped or lambda-shaped cracking. If the patient is experiencing dryness of the mouth, it is possible that blood will appear in the stool, and the patient will have small amounts of urine that is reddish in color, and stomach pains. If there is a spiked appearance on the tongue, the patient may suffer a possible liver and gall problem. If tongue is red and cracked, a lung and stomach problem is possible.

A red spot on the tip of the tongue signifies that the patient has been overworked and may be experiencing insomnia and stress. This symptom reveals that this patient is suffering from a deficiency of vitamins and nutrients.

If both sides of the tongue become red, this patient suffers from high blood pressure and a hyperactive thyroid gland.

If the symptoms are more extreme and the tongue darker in

color, besides being possibly an acute bacterial infection or chronic disease, like tuberculosis or hyperthyroid and cancers, these patients may have dilated capillary blood vessels, causing inflammation leading to a thickening of blood, resulting in slow moving blood.

If the tongue is PURPLE

This color on the tongue turns out to be an extreme case of tongue redness. Blood stasis causes the color change from red to purple. This could be due to a number of possibilities:

- Heart disease with lung infection, where the lung function is impaired, and thus the oxygen exchange process blocked.
- Fever symptoms due to unsaturated hemoglobin and high blood viscosity; the patient most likely suffers from poor circulation.
- Red blood cells are denser when ill, there is oxygen depletion causing an irregularity in blood density and production, causing a green purple color. This problem is also seen in alcohol poisoning.
- Early stages of circulation problems; cold temperatures and surroundings.

Internal trauma may also be the cause for purple or blue spots to appear on the tongue, as opposed to the whole tongue being a certain color.

If the tongue has been dark red or purple for a long time, this patient should immediately see a doctor about the possibility of preventing cancer. Out of 12,448 cancer patients, a majority of these patients were seen to have symptoms such as these, especially patients with esophageal and sphincter cancer. Leukemia and lung cancer patients also proved to have the same tongue symptoms as those mentioned above.

If the tongue appears to have a purple hue, this also could be caused by poor circulation in the patient's membrane vessels. This symptom may be caused by ailments such as chronic bronchitis, certain lung diseases, or heart failure diseases. One must understand that this color can also be a sign of gynecological and gastroenterological diseases. This purple hue may also be due to old age, as the blood tends to slow in old age.

A purple tongue body may also be due to a possibility that one or more hydrogens on a normally unreactive phenyl constituent in the bodily system has been replaced by a nitro or ammonium group, causing the binding with other unreactive substances and the formation of a purple color. People who work closely with pesticides, printing presses, plastics, textiles and/or explosives should be aware of this appearance.

If the tongue is GREEN

This hue has been shown to be mostly due to the later stages of a circulation problem. Reduction of hemoglobin amounts results in the overall lack of oxygen. The bodies veins become slow flowing and clogged due to the poor circulation and the blood will run with high viscosity and high counts of red blood cell. This condition is seen in patients suffering from alcoholism, pigment settlement, extremely cold temperatures, an increase in enzyme activity and blood clotting kinase activity, increased nitrates, pulmonary heart disease, liver sclerosis, hepatitis, coronary heart disease, gall bladder problems, edema, and uterine problems.

If the patient is a teenage girl and has green or light purple spots on the tip or the side of the tongue, then she suffers from irregular monthly cycles and/or painful menstruation or uterus bleeding. If the patient is an adult, this is a sign of blood stasis or of heart problems.

If the tongue sides have green/blue stripes, or if it is stiff, then this patient may be suffering from liver problems, and has the possibility of liver cancer.

If the tongue if BLACK

Patients are in their latest and most severe stages of disease if the tongue is black. The patient will have symptoms including shallow breathing, dizziness and heaviness of the head, the extremities will be cold and the pulse weak.

This color represents the final stages of disease if transgressed from yellow to gray to black. They are the most dangerous stages of physical disorder and infection (Pic. 4-d). At this stage, the kidney is in poor working condition, and both hot and cold characteristics are in the worst, most extreme conditions possible. The tongue is usually darkest at the back of the tongue, and lighter up front. Tongues that are black are usually fuzzy-looking, as if covered with mold.

Black, slimy, sticky palette:
The patient will be feverish, congested, have diarrhea and loose stool. These people generally do not like to drink water, and have cold chills throughout their bodies.

Black, dry palette:
This usually signals the extreme stages of lung disease; the kidney is very weak and debilitated. Yin and yang components of the character are both virtually empty by this stage The patient will feel immensely thirsty and nauseous, but be unable to vomit, as well as hot and feverish all over the body. She or he may be easily annoyed and have a weak pulse.

Black, dry, burnt-looking tongue with fuzzy growths, spikes or cracks:
These patients will feel constipated and terribly uncomfortable, as they are in their very last stages of disease. Other symptoms seen in patients include unclear, raspy voice and speech, thick, heavy breathing, and much heat throughout the body.

One must also check the coloring of the uncoated areas and the sides. Normally, the tongue is an even light-red color. But when the patient is ill, blood contents and concentration changes and the patient's tongue color will change accordingly.

Palette changes

How does one tell through tongue diagnosis if the patient is recovering? The tongue must be splotched before recovery, from thick to thin, from dense to very sparse, as a path to healing. Gradual recovery is the only true form of recovery until the new palette is entirely regrown. But if suddenly all the symptoms of disease are gone instantly, then the person's chi is seriously out of balance and the kidney is not functioning; this is definitely not the correct path of recovery.

10

Tongue Shape

Normally, the tongue is very flexible, supple, mobile, and not too thick or thin. In the case of a diseased patient, the patient's tongue varies in shape.

Teeth marks are the most important anomaly that can be immediately detected during diagnosis. These ridges along the sides of the tongue are due to the imprint of the teeth onto the tongue and are generally thought to be caused by water retention in the tongue (Pic. 3-c). Water retention can be due to spleen/pancreas problems, signaling need for improvement of the digestive system. If the spleen is bad, the kidney cannot work properly due to the interconnection between the two systems. Thus the excretory system does not function properly, and there is a retention of water that collects in the body, especially in the face and throat areas. The tongue is swollen due to this water retention, which forces it against the teeth, leaving teeth marks. Since the spleen has to do with immunity, and the pancreas controls much of digestion, this condition often leads to diabetes if left untreated for a period of time. This type of condition is commonly seen with the lack of lunulae on the nails, signaling poor circulation and oxygen saturation levels.

Patients are often prone to candidas infections and cancer; in fact, a majority (80%) of cancer patients have teeth marks and lack lunulae.

If the rim, the area around the edges of the tongue, is swollen, and the body of the tongue is puffy looking and has teeth marks on the side, then this person lacks protein. The tongue retains water due to the dearth of protein. Tongue tissue is generally more sensitive to water retention than other areas of the body. This accounts for the puffy appearance of the tongue.

If the tongue is so swollen that it hardly fits inside the mouth, then, if the patient happens to be a child, this is due to lowered thyroid functions. If the patient is an adult, this symptom could be due to the condition of the thyroid or pituitary gland. In the case of the pituitary gland, the anterior pituitary may become overly excited and release too many hormones. This excess amount of hormones causes swollen extremities as well as layer growth. A bloody red color signifies that the patient has liver cirrhosis.

Some patients may have tongues that bulge out in the front but are normal-sized the rest of the way back to the root, indicating hormonal imbalance as well as kidney problems that may derive from excess sexual activity or other habitual problems (Pic. 5-a).

If the tongue is thin and flat, this patient has poor circulation. If the tongue is white and flat, then this patient has poor circulatory and salivary functions. If the tongue is red and flat, then this patient's cardiovascular an digestive functions are poor. In the case of a truly chronic digestion problem, the patient should appear thin and suffer from a Yin and Yang deficiency.

Tongue Cracking

If the tongue has cracks, this is due to Vitamin B deficiency; chronic digestive problems; kidney, spleen and stomach are in poor condition.

This also refers to problems seen through noticing vertical or horizontal cracking or both, but if the problem is inherited, then these may not be related. Usually the lines appear directly related to stomach and spleen, the chi energy and metabolism is weak, and has poor absorption. Stomach, duodenal and cardiac sphincter cancer are all closely associated with the lines on the tongue. If the stomach seems to have problems and the lines are noticed to have arisen later on, then cancer is probable and should be checked.

Cracking down the center of the tongue toward the back is due to poor kidney function (Pic. 4-d). Cracking closer to the front of the tongue, down the center, is due to gastrointestinal or stomach problems and is also known as fissured tongue (Pic. 5-b) If there are cracks running horizontally across the tongue in the middle area, it may also be a kidney problem, and if there is a crack along the edges, this signals spleen dysfunction. These disorders can be improved with use of herbal products such as Asparagus Extract, Digestron and Vitamin B complex. Any crack over 2 mm deep should be considered a serious condition and given attention immediately. Also, the condition is serious if the tongue has an upside down T-shaped crack in it.

Tongue Pain

In the event of a vitamin B-12 deficiency, it is said that there will be pain felt in the tongue. This deficiency can be detected if the patient has the condition known as geographical tongue, and can be treated with vitamin supplements and Asparagus Extract. I should here issue a warning, however, concerning vitamin supplement usage: It has been discovered that folic acid supplements given to patients with a vitamin B-12 deficiency can lead to serious neurological damage. Thus, one must be sure of their vitamin deficiencies and body types before taking these vitamins. (Similar findings were also discovered concerning the excess of vitamins E, which will inhibit vitamin K functions and increase anti-thrombosis effects, and calcium, which inhibits iron and other trace element absorption.)

11

Coating

The coating of one's tongue can say a lot about the person's health, as well as whether or not their health is improving. There are two steps in determining the condition of one's coating:

1) Coating color
2) Coating description

A healthy person should have a thin, clear looking moisture film over their tongue. This film should not be too thick, too glossy, or too sticky.

Coating Color

A thick, yellow coating over the tongue is a sign that the patient has gastritis, digestion problems, or stomach ulcers. The darker the yellow, the more severe the condition.

A gray film coating the tongue in the root area may be caused by several types of bodily weaknesses such as frequent fevers, but are mostly due to kidney problems (Pic. 5-c), especially if the tongue is brown or black. If this symptom is not related to poor kidney functions, and the tongue still appears to be brown or black, then this may be a sign of trouble in the intestines and may be related to constipation. It may also be caused by overuse of broad spectrum antibiotics. Broad spectrum antibiotics kill the tongue's natural bacteria allowing fungus to grow and, thus, accounts for the dark brown or black film over the tongue.

If a patient notices a black film over his tongue that is present only in the mornings, he should not worry. The patient may experience frequent fevers that arise from ailments such as stomach, lung, or esophagus cancer. A patient who is highly nervous can also acquire symptoms such as these. If the root of the tongue is covered with a spiky, fur-like substance, then he patient is over-stressed and needs to relieve his tension. The yellow-brown film covering the tongue can also due to kidney-related hormone problems such as impotence, especially if there are red star-like spots on the tongue anywhere besides the tip. Later stages of this problem may turn black (Pic. 5-c).

If the coating of the tongue appears to be white and thick at first, then yellow, then brown, and finally black, then one has an extreme illness which should be examined immediately. If the color of the tongue appears to be changing from black to white, this signifies that one's health is improving.

If the tongue has no coating, this signifies that the patient is lacking protein and is often cold because he does not have enough fluid. If the tongue appears to be a purple color then the patient must avoid becoming septicemia. If the patient is elderly and has thick blood vessels, this signifies that the patient has cardiopulmonary disease.

Description of Coating

If the film over the tongue appears to be slippery, thick, and shiny, then this patient is often cold and is able to contract edemas easily. Patients with these symptoms may very well be suffering from bronchitis, asthma, or emphysema.

Yellow-white spots in the coating of the tongue signifies that the patient has poor digestion and has insufficient salivary glands. If a patient used to have a coating over the tongue but the coating seems to have dried up, then this patient is suffering from stomach problems.

If the tongue is covered with little white chunks and appears to be greasy, then the patient is suffering from a respiratory problem (Pic. 5-d). For this condition, it is helpful to use Synergen and MIT (See Appendix A).

If the tongue appears to be spiky, then this person's body gives off heat. This type of person does not eat well and is often a victim of fever or pneumonia. If the patient eats rough food, such as sugar cane, the tongue's lingual papillae (coating) will be irritated and will form tiny spikes.

If the coating of the tongue resemble the petals of a flower and has a thick coating, then the patient is suffering from a severe cold and an epidemic problem can arise.

Tiny spikes covering the tongue signifies that this patient has been suffering from scarlet fever for many days.

A wrinkled tongue with no coating signifies that the patient has liver problems.

If the tongue is covered with a frosty fur-like substance, this is due to poor spleen and pancreas functions as well as digestive problems. Digestron can be used here for beneficial results. (See Appendix A)

The patchy-looking geographical tongue, named after the map-like appearance of the tongue due to loss of coating in certain areas, has two types that relate to different problems. One type of appearance, in which there is a light, thin white patchy coating indicates respiratory, allergies, or sinus problems, and can be related to parasites in the body (Pic. 6-a). If the geographical tongue also shows cracking, with deeper cracks being up to 2-3 mm deep and a yellow coating, this second type is due to a digestion problem. This type of tongue coating may be caused by stomach and pancreas problems (Pic. 6-b). The worst for both cases is if there is no coating in the root or back of the tongue, and is mainly in the middle of the tongue. This indicates a more serious condition. If the coating is only on one side, this is intermediate condition. Geographical tongue also can be helped by vitamin B-12, thiamin, and folic acid supplements in conjunction with Synergen for the first type and Asparagus and Digestron for the second type.

12

Thickness, Moisture, and the Underside

A healthy person should have a medium-thin tongue that is lightly coated by a white film. The tongue should be large enough to fit soundly into the area between all the teeth, but no larger or smaller than that. If the tongue is small in appearance and is very thin, that signifies that the patient is very weak. If the tongue is very thick is covered with a fur-like film, that signifies that the patient is prone to illnesses although physically strong.

A healthy person excretes just enough saliva so that the tongue is always moist. A patient's insufficient amount of saliva secretion may be caused by not enough fluid intake or absorption. For instance, when a patient has diarrhea, the patient's body tongue will appear to have a very dry and rough surface. Another cause of insufficient saliva secretion can be related to high fevers. When a patient's body temperature rises, the fluids in its system become used up so the saliva glands secrete only a small amount of saliva to conserve the body's water content.

Western medicine also takes note of the condition of the

tongue. If a patient suffers from a severe case of constipation, diarrhea, or poor digestion, the tongue will appear greasy and swollen. If a patient usually feels bloated, has diarrhea, and has a lack of coating over the tongue, this signifies that the patient has eaten too many oily foods and is now experiencing an upset stomach. A patient with these symptoms should relax and fast for a while until the symptoms subside.

If a patient wakes up in the morning with a thick tongue but gradually reduces after the patient's daily habits, there is no need to worry. If the coating over the tongue becomes thicker over the day's routine, this means that the illness is spreading deeper into the body. Another sign that the illness is spreading is if the mouth becomes very dry and the salivary glands cannot secrete enough saliva to keep the mouth moist. Recovery paths can be identified when the tongue turns from thick to thin, from dark to light, and from dry to moist.

If the tongue is swollen, marked and very moist, slippery with side teethmarks caused by swelling of the tongue, these are all signs of spleen problems. The reason for this swelling is due to the edema of the tongue tissue that is caused by water retention in the area. But there are some holistic doctors who feel that this swelling can be related to poor digestive functions, and if one looks at the diagram of the 5 elements and 5 main organ systems, it is easily seen that indeed there is the possibility of a connection between spleen function and digestive function, thus explaining the slightly varying interpretations of the condition.

Underside of the Tongue

The two veins found on the underside of the tongue are connected mainly to heart and liver functions. Build-up of any kind has been found to be easily seen under the tongue. So any change of blood vessel consistency or change of color can be correlated to a change of bodily function.

If the two veins on the underside of a person's tongue are not light pink or blue but dark red or purple and protruding out like varicose veins, then the patient has very poor circulation. This type of condition, along with the presence of red or black dots or a spider vein-like appearance, is indicative of heavy metal accumulation in the system. Heavy metals like lead, most commonly found in tap water and paint, and mercury, found in the amalgam dental fillings for cavities, as well as aluminum and cadmium, found in cooking utensils or cans and hair dye, respectively, are common contributors to heart diseases and mental disorders. These toxins, though encountered in everyday life, in forms such as car exhaust and pollution, are potentially dangerous and must be removed from the system. If the veins on the underside of the tongue branch out and spread, a liver problem can be detected and thus these people have trouble detoxifying. This would account for the indication of heavy metals under the tongue (Pic. 4-c,d). Thus, for everyone with liver problems, there is a heavy metal accumulation due to the decreased ability to detoxify the system. However, the same cannot be said vice versa, for not everyone with heavy metal accumulation has a liver problem.

Clinically, we can see that diseased patients have different appearances on the underside of the tongue in terms of size and shading of the main blood vessels that branch from the base of the mouth, where the tongue is attached. If there is any color deviation from the normal red color of blood vessels, this may indicate a problem in oxygen uptake by blood and a pH deviation in blood. The patient may have TB, chronic bronchitis, emphysema, hypertension or kidney/heart problems. The factors in the diagnosis of the tongue are the fleshiness of the tongue itself, the palette appearance, tongue form, and tongue movement.

Characteristics such as puffy, bloated looking veins under the tongue of blue purple, purple green, or purple black colorings indicate heavy metal poisoning due to environmental pollutants such as car exhaust and smog, as well as such toxins as hair dye and amalgam tooth fillings, all of which contain heavy metals. If such color exists but is rather light, this indicates that the poisoning is still in its early stages. This will cause restlessness and annoyance, difficulty in swallowing, with lots of phlegm. The more noticeable the discoloration, the more extreme the condition and the greater the need for oral chelation and detoxification. Vein Lite has been used quite successfully in both Japan and the United States for oral chelation, increasing blood circulation, and detoxification of blood.

13

Tongue Diagnosis by System

Using these examining outlines, one should be able to, with practice, learn to correlate the appearance of the tongue to problems in the body. Tongue diagnosis results are grouped into the 5 main systems of the body below, so that one can confirm the correct general conditions upon checking the following categories:

Lung Problems:

If the patient has pulmonary and/or respiratory problems, the area of the tongue on the side just behind the tip will be red or spotted like a strawberry, with a thin, white coating and/or bulging (Pic. 6-c). The front side of the tongue surface may be raised due to swelling or there may be detectable raised red points which are related to allergy, asthma, or bronchitis. The pulse felt will be faint. Other symptoms include fever, aversion to cold, coughs, and headaches, and calls for a reduction of heat and improvement of the respiration and oxygen levels, a problem that can be improved by taking Synergen and MIT.

Liver Problems:

Liver problems leave the tongue dark-red with bruised edges and a dark or grey coating (Pic. 6-d,7-a). One should also look underneath the tongue for branched veins (Pic. 7-b). If the liver function is bad, there is a detoxification problem and poisons and heavy metals are allowed to be left in the body. People with liver disorders tend to have bloated stomachs, dry mouths with a generally bitter taste. Other symptoms include heart problems and a general feeling of warm discomfort. Dizziness and confused thinking may also be present. Treatment calls for the adjustment of liver functions and detoxification (of such toxins as heavy metals, etc.) by use of Liver Chi (See Appendix A).

Heart Problems:

Generally, problems of the heart can be detected by looking at the tip of the tongue, which will appear thin and red, and sometimes elongated (Pic. 7-c,d). If the tip of the tongue is especially red with dark spots, this shows a heart problem such as pulmonary heart disease or coronary heart disease (Pic. 8-a,b,c). The tip of the tongue may also have a white coating accompanied by a faint pulse. Heart and artery problems can also be indicated by a purple-red, stiff tongue with little to no overall coating and a mirror-like, dry look. The pulse may be faint, even when felt under some amount of pressure. Other symptoms include fever, perspiration, thirst, dizziness, aversion to cold, coughs, confusion, joint pain and headaches. This condition requires detoxification of bodily toxins (including heavy metals, etc.) and calls for a reduction of heat and improvement of respiration and oxygen levels, as circulation decreases with the effects. Vein

Lite is an excellent product of choice for these symptoms, for its oral chelative properties and ability to increase blood circulation.

Digestion- Stomach/Spleen Problems:

If the patient has stomach or digestive problems, the tongue will be thick and yellow with a spiky coating and she or he will have an overall dry mouth. The pulse will be strong, and other symptoms may include fever, perspiration, chest congestion, wheezing, rash, and constipation. This problem calls for the reduction of heat and excretion of waste, by taking the herbal product Digestron.

Problems of the spleen leave the tongue a purple-reddish color, with a thick, yellowish coating that has a greasy look (Pic. 8-b). Most importantly is the presence of teeth marks which will indicate spleen problems. (Pic. 3-c) The pulse will be felt upon medium pressure, and the other symptoms include congestion, vomiting, heat, and a urinary condition where there is only concentrated, small amounts of urine. Treatment calls for use of a diuretic and the reduction of heat, effectively accomplished by taking Asparagus Extract. Digestron will also help in spleen function and overall digestion.

Kidney/Hormone Problems:

Poor kidney function causes the tongue to be light red and the coating thin and dry, especially in the root area which will turn from yellow to black. The pulse felt will be faint, and the body and face will feel hot with a ruddy complexion. Other symptoms may include fatigue, and hot palms and feet. Treatment calls for improvement of the kidney/hormone balance and cleansing of the blood, through use of Chi Energy and Vein Lite. Kidney function is also related to hormonal balance, and problems with the kidney often indicate an imbalance in bodily hormones. Chi Energy has been effectively used to rebalance the levels of hormones and their output and usage in the body (Pic. 8-d and Appendix A). Star-like red spots on the tongue is indicative of hormonal imbalance which could be female, male and thyroid hormones. Sometimes also, the fingernails will have white spots to support this indication. This condition in teens is all right since they are in developmental stages, but for a grown male this could signal impotence or prostate problems, while for female it is definitely a hormonal imbalance. Use MIT to treat the lower back and abdominal areas for this condition, and Myomin can also help for female organs. For males, use MIT on the lower back and perineum area.

Most people take estrogen or progesterone, or even DHEA, but how do you know that your hormones are truly balanced upon taking these medications? Here, you can use our Ovuscope kit to check your hormone balance everyday, which can prove very convenient as well as economic (see Appendix A on the Ovuscope.)

14

Diagnostic Kit for Nail and Tongue Examination

My preventative diagnostic kit is currently being widely used to quickly diagnose one's general condition by simply looking at the presence or absence of lunulae on the fingernail and the teethmarks on the tongue. It is the result of the 10,000 cancer patient cases I have reviewed under my father's guidance, in which I have found similar and distinct markers in the lunulae and teethmarks, allowing me to categorize the general conditions based on these visual markers into 7 different, abnormal groups. It then gives the correlative symptoms and suggestions for treatment using herbs and other natural remedies. The following is a comprehensive overview of the diagnostic kit, which I first introduced to the public in 1994 as a way to detect problems before CT scans or blood tests come back, before problems worsen.

To use the disc, one first finds an appropriate description of the person to be tested on the outer disc or disc B. Once the person's outward fingernail appearance has been found, turn the inner disc or disc A so that the color or the characteristic matches on both discs. The corresponding tongue description should match the person's characteristics as a confirmation. Now read the paragraphs beneath the disc A cutaway opening onto the outer disc for possible symptoms and directions for improvement. If one has more than about 50% of the symptoms listed, then he or she is probably in the right category of description, as not everyone will have *all* the symptoms listed.

Nail matrices take about 3 months to grow up to the point of regular nail growth, and then one must allow another 6-8 months (in adults) for complete nail growth. A normal, healthy person should have 8 lunulae; four on each fingernail and none on the pinkies. Lack thereof indicates poor intracellular oxygen levels, and can lead to symptoms such as cold hands and feet, numbness, memory loss, and fatigue. In this condition, the patient may have higher risk of cancer and candidas yeast infection. If one hand has less or smaller lunulae than the other, then this indicates a circulation blockage on that side of the body. Lack of lunulae with no markings on the tongue signal cardiovascular problems.

There should be no teethmarks on the edge of the tongue. Teethmarks indicate problems in the spleen and pancreas. Spleen function is related to the immune system, while pancreas function is necessary for digestion. Teethmarks on the tongue can indicate the possibility of diabetes, especially if it already runs in the family. If both markers are present (teethmarks and lack of lunulae), then the patient is in what I hypothesize to be the high risk category for cancer. If the oxygen saturation is low, and immunity is low, then cancer has the chance to invade. Also, if it is already in the family medical history, the patient must be especially careful. If the thumb has lunulae only, and there are teethmarks on the tongue, the patient may already have early stages of cancer, which may not yet be detectable by other tests. In fact, by the time blood tests or CT scans can detect cancer, it may already be in later stages and difficult to stop. Teethmarks on the inner cheek can also be of this indication.

There are also three different groups of abnormality which can be described as the cold group, the hot group, and the hot/cold mixed group. Each of these three main categories also has beneath them three subcategories to speak of:

If the lunulae are barely noticeable, smaller than 1-2 mm, or if there are less than eight on both hands (between 3 and 7), this person is considered to be of the cold type. These people are also likely to have teethmarks on the tongue and inner cheek if the condition is extreme. She or he will often feel very cold, like warm climate and foods, and have occasional poor digestion. This condition calls for some fresh ginger in the diet and red, or fermented, tea along with Vein Lite, Asparagus Extract, Chi Energy, and Fibre-Cleanse.

If the patient has lunulae only on the thumbs, they are in a more extreme cold condition and will most likely have teethmarks along the edge of the tongue and the inner cheek. She or he will feel weak, drowsy, cold in the extremities, have poor digestion and low immunity. This situation calls for a diet rich in fresh ginger, warm, spicy foods, along with Vein Lite, Asparagus Extract, and Chi Energy.

Patients that have no lunulae at all are in the most severely poor condition and are considered to the extremely cold types. These patients are at a high risk for cancer, and will often have very pronounced teethmarks on the tongue and inner cheek. They will appear sallow-complexioned and pale, weak and may be overweight. They may experience insomnia and excessive dreaming, low immunity, the frequent need to urinate, cold extremities and poor digestion with loose stool. Females may have severe menstrual cramps and heavy discharge; other symptoms include chronic sinusitis, oral hygiene problems, gastroenteritis, hepatitis, and renalitis. These patients are highly recommended to take fresh ginger, red tea, spicy foods, Asparagus Extract, Vein Lite, Chi Energy, Slender All, and use the Mineral Infrared Device.

Patients that have large lunulae but with unclear, hazy boundaries may often feel hot in their torso area but cold elsewhere (Pic. 1-d). This mixed bodily type is a combination of both Hot and Cold types and is referred to on my kit as the Hot/Cold Mixed Group. People in this group stem from Hot characteristics and become more cold upon insufficient care of their bodies. There are three stages to this condition. In its early stage, the boundary between the lunulae and the flesh of the finger tip begins to cloud up, but is not conspicuous and may even be like the slightly Hot category. It is best if one prevents this stage from getting worse if it is caught this early on. Cold has only partially entered the body, so it may not be easily noticed. In the middle stages, the boundary between the lunulae and the flesh has become quite hazy, and the person may feel coldness in the extremities as the Cold moves in even more. Teethmarks are here beginning to show. In the final stages of the mixed group, the lunulae are barely distinguishable from the flesh on the fingertip beneath the nail, and the Cold has now claimed a majority of the body. The Cold may even have spread to the kidneys and all over the torso. It is at this dire point that cancer can grow, and spread very quickly. To prevent this, care must be taken early on, and the early stage of the condition calls for lots of fresh fruit in the diet, Chi Energy or Asparagus Extract.

If the patient has small lunulae on every nail on the hands including the pinkies, or even if one hand has fewer than the correct number of lunulae while the other has a lunulus on the pinky, she or he is considered to be in the hot category, in which there are three subcategories. In the slightly hot subcategory, the patient is in overall good health, but may also experience dryness in the mouth, occasional dizziness, constipation and poor digestion. Fruits and vegetables are in order here, along with a decrease in the amount of spicy foods eaten. Patients should also take Cymosi Fibre-Cleanse, Asparagus Extract, Vein Lite, and Diabend if necessary.

If the patient has rather large lunulae on the nails, or more than 8 lunulae total, he or she is considered to the hot, and may feel anxious, restless, and experience dry mouth often, along with dizziness and constipation. These patients should not eat spicy foods and should eat more fruits and vegetables, and take green tea with Vein Lite, Cymosi Fibre-Cleanse, and Diabend.

If there are large lunulae on all the fingernails, this person is in an extreme physical condition called the very hot category on my kit and will have other symptoms such as redness of the face, high energy to the point of hyperactivity, a loud voice and a big temper. These people definitely need to eat plenty of fruits and vegetables, take green tea, and take Vein Lite, Diabend, and Cymosi Fibre-Cleanse.

It is apparent through reviewing cancer patient files that approximately 80% of all cancer patients are of the cold category of varying degrees. This does not mean that only those in the cold category are at a risk of this disease, nor does it guarantee that hot types never get cancer. Of course, there are deviations. However, this does not say that cold types are generally at a higher risk of cancer than hot types, and thus care must be taken to prevent it from happening.

I will here clarify that even if the rest of the fingernails have no lunulae, if there are lunulae on the pinkies, then this still indicates heart problems. One does not necessarily have to have a Hot condition to have heart problems; Cold types often have them also.

Part III

Confirmation Using Other Diagnostic Techniques

This section is dedicated to explaining how to confirm the results of one method of analysis by using another method. For instance, if a person wished to confirm that the results from the tongue and nail diagnosis paralleled those from another methods of analysis, such as hair loss analysis, she could easily check the symptoms by referring to the below chapter of information. The following pages are dedicated to the confirmation of the results attained by fingernail and tongue diagnosis using several different physical markers on the body, and produced by the body:

Biological Clocks

To test one's health, it often ept to use examine one's biological clock, to look at her or his bodily rhythms. Melatonin is one of these adjuster of a biological clock.

What exactly is a biological clock? On earth, every species has a rhythm by which members of that group live their lives, in a cycle controlled in a time-clock manner. This is called their biological clock. Even humans, who are the most recently evolved species, are controlled by this clock. Our bodily functions and substance levels are maintained via internal and external factors. Everything from your pulse to your behavior can be regulated by the biological clock. An example of this is a woman's monthly menstrual cycle, during which her uterine and vaginal linings, mucous membranes, body temp, secretions, and many other things, are changing in response to her cycle.

Human moods and stability correlate to the body's immunity level. The more stable a person's moods, the higher immunity that individual enjoys. Similarly, certain times of a day relate to a strengthened or weakened immune response. This can affect the symptoms of different diseases. In rheumatoid fever, the fevers tend to get worse in the evening. Similarly for bronchitis and asthma, the coughing and symptoms tend to worsen as night sets. In this way, diseases are also affected by the biological clock.

Endocrinologists find that patients suffering from hyper adrenocorticosteroid function tend to have less problems in the daytime and more at night. Hence, doctors must be aware of the proper time to take a blood test for different diseases.

Coronary heart disease is at is worst in the early morning, a point that I shall refer to as its "peak". Heart attacks peak at mid-morning, cardiac arrest in the early morning as well. At these peaks, the death rates for these diseases are at their highest.

In the morning, diabetes is at its worst and the anti-insulin hormone is at its highest level, thus the patient's blood sugar will be very high and most serious in the morning. Rheumatoid pain is also high at this time. Understanding one's biological clock can help one prepare for these peaks and alleviate the symptoms.

Scientists have learned of over 100 different rhythms in the body. There are daily, monthly, seasonal, and even annual rhythms. Also, research has found that the body's natural rhythm controls mainly three areas of bodily function:

1)energy, 2)mood, and 3)intellect. Each person has a cycle upon birth for each of these main groups. The cycle for bodily energy goes once every 23 days. Moods and temper cycle once every 28 days, and the intellect cycles once every 33 days. At the point on the cycle that all 3 points are at their highest, one will feel their best and most energetic, with acute memory and stable moods. It is said that the midpoints between these cycles are the points where there is the most danger of contracting diseases, or for diseases to get worse. One can determine the point they are at on their biological cycle by assuming that when they are born, they are at the midpoint of the sine-wave-like cycle just before the incline to the maximum. Then all you need to do is divide the amount of days you've been alive by the length of each specific cycle to find out where you are on it.

Ancient saying goes that one should get up with the sunrise to start working and go to bed upon sunset. There is logic to these rituals. Biological clock specialists note that people's bodies are like clocks. Behavior is precisely regulated according to these clocks, and any deviation will result in serious problems. Chronobiology experts say that besides the 5 senses, we also have a sense of time that our biological clock runs on. The liver, small intestines, mucous membranes all have specific functions; even the smallest cells have time-related functions.

The most sensitive organ to the time sense is by far the brain. The brain's biological clock function allows for regular, restful sleep, as well as vigorous thought and exercise drive and motivation. Even one's appetite is controlled, via brain function, by a biological clock. In a society where everyone has professional and social obligations, so every one is following their watches. This is the price of modernization of our society, the need to synchronize. The best time to think is about 10 am, when your alertness is peaking and short term memory is at its strongest. So meetings during which brainstorming is necessary will most productively occur at this hour. Many people need vacations in summer, but actually the body is most relaxed annually toward the end of February. Hence the coming of the Chinese New Year brings with it a time of rest and relaxation, as it happens at the end of February on the Western Calendar.

Hair

As many people are already aware, the purpose of hair is not only to provide protection to the scalp. Hair accurately reflects the status of your health. It is made of corneal protein, 10 trace elements, and has more than 20 amino acids and derivatives, including zinc, iron, and copper. Measuring trace elements helps to reveal disease symptoms. Hair and other constituents have continued metabolism.

There are around 100,000 hairs on every adult head. Each hair usually lasts 3-4 years, and grows 0.2-0.3 mm per day. Normally, 90% of an adult's hair is growing while 10% is falling out. An average adult loses 60-100 hairs a day, but because an adult normally has an abundance of hair, this daily loss of hair usually goes unnoticed. If a person loses more than 100 hairs a day, the hair loss will soon become apparent and the person will be experiencing a balding effect.

Reasons for balding include:
1) Physical instability-pregnant or post-partum
2) Pathological diseases-pneumonia, tinea, anemia, tumor
3) Genetically inherited baldness

Hair growth and loss of hair is related to problems with the patient's kidney system. Energetic people with healthy hair usually have strong kidney systems. A person with good kidney function will have strong and healthy hair. If the kidney function is not good, on the other hand, then the hair will turn white earlier and the person will age quicker overall. If white hair appears and the patient is not too old, the problem may be either genetic or of nervous origins, or it may be due to disease such as tuberculosis, digestive problems, anemia, and atherosclerosis. If hair that is not naturally dark turns dark suddenly, then it could be due to such extreme conditions as melanoma. If the person's hair is falling out, it could be due to a deficiency in zinc. If hair is brittle and easily broken, this is indicative of a thyroid problem. If there is relatively little hair and the hair is dry and shriveled-looking, then the kidney system needs to be repaired. Hair loss in men is commonly correlated to poor kidney function, and in women this is organ deficiency is indicated by similar balding or patchiness.

Hair loss at the top of the head may be due to cholic problems, those relating to the gall bladder and bile. If there is bodily hair loss as well as balding, this may be indicative of a hormonal imbalance. Anytime hair seems to fall out more readily than normal, or is hair loss is noticed, one should be aware of possible problems associated to the condition.

As males reach adulthood, if the scalp becomes oilier, with a tendency to result in dandruff, this may also be a sign of possible future hair loss.

Eyebrows

Eyebrows function to protect the eyes from sweat and dust in the area, trapping particles before they can enter and irritate. Darker colored eyebrows signify healthy and strong kidney function. But if the eyebrow hairs are sparse over the area and lighter in color than the rest of the body's hair, there may be a variety of possible associations to this:
1) there could be adhesive tissue edema
2) anterior pituitary function may be down
3) there may be thyroid dysfunction or decreased activity.

One way to test for thyroid function is to stand erect and allow your arms to fall loosely at your side. If your palms naturally turn inward, that is normal. However, if the palms instead turn and face our beyond the rear of the body, then that is indicative of a thyroid problem. Another way is to look at the three middle fingers of your most frequently used hand. The ring finger, or fourth finger, should be longer than the pointer, or second finger. If this is not the case, then there may be a thyroid condition.

If the eyebrow hairs stand upright instead of laying against the skin, and are dry feeling, this would signal either a nervous system condition, or the case of certain women, a menstrual condition. Women with particularly dark eyebrows may have high levels of adrenocortico steroids in their system.

Face Color

A person's general facial overtones can say a lot about their health. Eyes should be clear and bright. Even if the patient has an acute condition yet still has a nice-colored complexion and clear eyes, the condition is in a stage optimistic for improvement. But if the face color has no vitality and is ruddy and dark in complexion, along with having bright eyes and being energetic, then the disease is probably chronic and much harder to cure.

If the face has a greenish color, then the patient may have a liver problem. If the face is reddish, then the patient has a heart problem. If the face is yellowish, then there is a stomach and pancreas problem. If the face is a pale white, then there could be a lung problem. A blackish complexion signals a kidney problem.

In more detail, the following can be said about a person with a reddish complexion: possible high blood pressure, high rates of fever, possibility of tuberculosis. These patients may exhibit symptoms of lupus such as the typical butterfly-shaped patch on the lower cheeks. Any other patch-like appearance on the lower cheek will signal a heart problem.

There are several reasons why one would have a yellowish complexion:
1) If the patient eats vegetables, certain types may invoke a yellowish appearance upon digestion which should return to normal after a while.
2) If not caused by the pigments in vegetables, it could be

jaundice, which is due to hepatitis, which can be detected by looking at the eyes to see if the whites of the eye are yellow in color along with the rest of the body.

Eyes

Poor eyesight is sometimes attributable to a deficiency in vitamin B and vitamin A. If a person is middle-aged, and suddenly has poor eyesight, then it could be due to diabetes.

If one is far-sighted due to old age, but suddenly feels that she or he is able to see better for a temporary period of time, this could be due to an onset of cataracts. Cataracts cause initial swelling of the lenses, so that eyesight is temporarily repaired.

If one can not see well at night, it is due to a lack of retinal, or vitamin A, which works the rod function of nighttime vision.

Sclera

Sclera, the whites of the eye, should be unspotted and totally white. Any deviation from this normal color and quality could indicate a problem:

Pregnant women, or children, who exhibit sclera coated with a blue tint may suffer from anemia. Sclera that are covered with green spots indicate that the patient has poor liver functions.

Patients who have yellow, jaundiced sclera suffer from liver or bile duct dysfunction. Sclera that appears to be jaundiced may be due to blood hemolysis.

Broken blood vessels that cover the sclera are often due to atherosclerosis and problems with the arteries in the brain.

Small, red spots covering the sclera are the result of broken capillaries and dilation.

Pinkeye infection, a temporary infection caused by the diseases contracted from unsanitary conditions, is characterized by itching and irritation in the area along with redness of the area.

Redness in the sclera can also be due to insomnia and poor sleeping habits. A person with poor heart functions and hypertension may also exhibit redness in the sclera. These symptoms, such as hypertension, are precursors to more serious ailments such as strokes.

Redness in only one eye can be attributed to the fact that the patient may suffer from certain infection including genital infections.

Sclera that appear to be coated with blue or grey dots are often causes by problems in the intestines such as tapeworms.

Iris

If the milky, white ring encircling the iris becomes red, then the eyes are characterized to be sensitive to sunlight. A patient with these symptoms may experience pain, blurred vision, and an occasional secretion of tears. These symptoms may also be the cause of iritis, the inflammation of the iris.

Shiny, green rings encircling the iris may be due to poor liver functions or copper accumulation. Copper accumulation is very damaging to the system for copper is an extremely toxic substance.

A white ring around the iris suggests that the patient suffers from high cholesterol levels. These symptoms may also be obvious in youngsters as well as adults. This symptoms may indicate that the person has brain atherosclerosis or certain heart diseases.

If the entire iris has a white layer over it and is cloudy, then it could be due to cataracts. Pain in the eyes and headaches, along with nausea, could be due to glaucoma.

If any of these abnormalities are seen and they could possibly spread or worsen as time goes on, it is important to go to a physician to check on it immediately.

Pupil

The average pupil is about 2.5mm in size in regular indoor lighting. Pupils, however, will dilate in lower light in order to get a better image of the view in focus. Similarly, in bright light, pupils will adjust to a small diameter in order to allow for less light to enter the eye.

Patients who have pupils that are less than 1.5mm in diameter often suffer from poor responses to light and dilation wounds of the pupil. The dilation wounds can be related to recent experience of a concussion or meningitis.

Small pupils are often due to alcohol poisoning, irritation due to certain sleeping pills, and hemorrhaging. Small pupils can also be due to organic phosphate or morphine poisoning. Patients with these symptoms are also prone to tumor growths.

Two pupils that are different in sizes can often be due to spinal tuberculosis or syphilis.

Pupils that appear to be very cloudy and white indicate that the patient has cataracts. These symptoms can also suggest that the patient suffers from glaucoma, a very strong case of myopia, or diabetes. (Cataracts is the number one reason for the loss of vision in the world.)

Pupils that exhibit a yellow hue signify that the patient may have retinoblastoma. If the patient happens to be a child of 7 or 8 years of age, then retinoblastoma most likely has been genetically transferred.

Green pupils signify that the patient suffers from glaucoma and pains in the eye.

Eye color is due to racial variety and genetics. If the surface of the iris is covered with bright dots, then there is a problem with the nerves in the brain.

The left eye generally reflects the condition of the right side of the body. The right eye reflects the condition of the left side of the body. This method of diagnosis is most accurate (80%) for the detection of angina pain, cholinitis, and duodenal ulcers. Bodily symptoms cause pain and spots that correlate on the eyes.

Bulging Eyes

If one eye appears to bulge, this means that the patient has a brain tumor which is pushing out within the skull. If both eyes bulge, this signifies that the patient suffers from hyperthyroid and fast heart palpitation. Bright eyes may indicate thyroid swelling. Other causes of this symptoms may be due to high blood pressure, Parkinson's disease, leukemia, hemophilia, or the lack of Vitamin B or D.

Sunken Eyes

Patients who have sunken eyes are usually thin, emotionally upset, choleric and have malaria, diarrhea, or diabetes. If eyes lack energy, the pupils would dilate and the entire face would turn grey.

Eyeballs that are dry and without luster are generally Vitamin A deficient. Patients with these symptoms often result in blindness. Dark circles under the eye suggest that the person suffers from the lack of enough sleep. If the area around the eyes are completely dark, then this patient has a serious kidney and circulatory problem. A person may also have adreno-cortico steroids dysfunction or cardiovascular microcirculation problem.

Puffiness underneath the eyes indicate that the patient has

not had enough sleep. He may be suffering from heart diseases or renalitis.

Droopy eyelids often suggest that the patient suffers from a Vitamin B1 deficiency, brain vessel problems, or poor energy.

Pale yellow patches on the upper corner of the eyebrow signify that the person's blood lipid levels are high. (An interesting thing to note in this type of examination is that, by examining Da Vinci's "Mona Lisa," one can see that the subject of the painting, because of the obvious portrayal of yellow patches on the eyebrow, actually had heart disease.)

Ears

Clinically, the ear has the most pressure points so any symptoms that the body shows will be recognized on the ear, changes will appear. There is a problem if the ear thickens or if a bump is felt. Ear canal lump growth can be due to lung, liver or spleen. Clinically, it is found that the outer ear has the most to do with lungs. If the ear is thick or has lumps, then it follows that lips and nails are purple. If the tongue has purple markings inside or the underside is bloated, in cancer patients it will signify an extreme condition, the ear changes slowly.

Over the years, the relationship between the ear and the body has been studied by many doctors around the world. Recent studies have shown that the larger the size of the ear, the healthier the person. Big earlobes signify a healthy kidney and body. The skin around the ears should be smooth and supple, not dipped or bumpy in anyway. For instance, patients who have liver cirrhosis have a knot in the center of their inner ear. Bumps in the lower inner ear may suggest that the patient suffers from chronic bronchitis. If the lining of the outer ear has ridges or bumps, then the person may have a bone spur or pains in the neck area.

A diagonal line across the earlobe, as well as wrinkles in both ears, indicates that the person has coronary heart disease. Patients who have this thin, diagonal line have a markedly high death rate. Within eight years, 75% of the patients tested with this line die, whereas only 57% without this line die. If the ears contain visible blood vessels, then this patient has heart diseases such as myocardial infarctions, coronary heart disease, or coronary dilation weakness or incapacity. Thin earlobes usually suggest that the patient has poor kidney functions or diabetic problems.

Nose

If the tip of the nose is very hard, then the patient suffers from atherosclerosis or high levels of cholesterol. A swollen tip often means that the person has a problem with his pancreas or kidney. If the nose is totally swollen and large, then the heart of the patient is also enlarged. French doctors have observed and studied over 2000 cancer cases and have discovered that patients who have aquiline shaped noses have the highest chance of acquiring lung cancer and laryngitis; patients with flat noses run the greatest risk of growing lymphatic tumors; patients with large noses have the greatest chance of getting pancreas or colon cancer; and patients with sharp, well-defined noses have the highest chance to acquire liver or breast cancer.

Although repeated shown through many test cases, these statistics are not 100% accurate.

If the inside of the nose is rough, this patient is unhealthy, for a variety of reasons ranging from chronic colds to prolonged drug abuse to respiratory infections.

If the barrier between the nostrils are rotted and rough-feeling, then this patient may have contracted syphilis.

A red appearance on the outside of the nose signifies that the person has digestive problems. If capillary blood vessels are apparent on the outside of the nose, then this person has a bacterial infection and may have had too much to drink.

Lips

Lips that are easily cut and rough could be related to a chronic stomach or intestinal problem. If the problem happens to occur in a newborn child, then this symptom is due to the fact that the baby has inherited syphilis. Dry or cracking corners of the mouth usually indicate that the patient has a membrane inflammation.

If the lips are always dry and cracked, this person may be dehydrated or unused to the weather. This person is Vitamin B deficient and lacks a diet rich with fresh fruits and vegetables.

Lip Color

Healthy lips should red, moist, and with a pale luster that is indicative of healthy habits and good blood circulation.

If both lips are pale or white, then this patient suffers from anemia or bleeding.

Greenish-white upper lips indicate that the person has a colon problem such as diarrhea or recurring stomach aches.

Pale lower lips often suggest that the patient has stomach problems such as vomiting, diarrhea, and minor pains.

Light pink or light red lips suggest that the patient is weak but not very ill.

Red, dark-colored lips suggest a fever or pulmonary heart disease. If the lips continue to grow darker and become the color of cherries, then this person has carbon monoxide poisoning.

If both lips are dark green or blue, then it is a circulatory problem and the patient should exhibit acute symptoms.

Completely dark lips suggest that the patient has a kidney problem. The darker the color of the lips, the more extreme the case. Dark lips can be attributed to insomnia, digestive problems, headaches, and a poor appetite.

Many lips have black spots due to chronic hypoadreno-cortico steroid output. If the corners of the mouth are black spotted, the patient has a poor digestive tract.

Inside of the Mouth

The inside of the mouth should be of a pink color. If the mouth is covered with blue or black spots then the patient has lowered adreno-cortico steroid. Blood spots usually suggest a Vitamin C deficiency. One should take note of red, white, or black patches.

White patches occur more easily in males. About 1-5% of these spots become cancerous. Smokers have more spots than the norm. These white patches are hardened and protruding, causing future lesions.

Red patches are softer, brighter, and not as painful as the white patches. These red patches usually occur on the tip of the tongue, underneath the tongue, or the bottom of the mouth. These patches are less likely to occur but have a greater chance of getting cancer.

Black patches generally grow on the roof of the mouth. Men have the patches more than women at a 2:1 ratio. Almost 30% of these patches will become cancerous. Patients exhibiting these symptoms should be aware of their health and take immediate precautions against the worsening of the condition to the point that it becomes cancerous.

Neck

The lymph nodes on the neck are very indicative of a person's health. It is also important to note the thyroid condition. If a person observes irregular sized knots that are under the skin, then the person suffers from a chronic inflammation of the lymph nodes. If the neck becomes red, painful, and hot, the person is experiencing an acute inflammation of the lymph nodes.

A swollen, bumpy, and uneven-faced neck is often indicative of thyroid tumors.

Body Weight

Waist circumference divided by hip circumference gives a number that is used by doctors commonly to show if the patient is overweight or underweight depending on their bodily fat content:
Men: 0.85-0.9 (fatter than average)
Women: 0.75-0.8

Causes for a person to appear over-thin:
1) poor appetite or digestive system
2) chronic insomnia and neurasthenia
3) chronic malnutrition
4) lack of enough exercise during bodily development.

It is important to understand that it is very unhealthy to be underweight. If a patient's digestive system has an ulcer, then the patient may appear to be thin. If this patient does not have an ulcer, her or his thinness may be due to cancer. An average person above 60 years of age is usually thinner then normal. This is okay, as it is a normally seen part of aging. The typical reasons for weight loss that the patient has not had enough nutrition or sleep. A patient's weight loss can also be due to chronic mild diarrhea, gastritis, or digestion ulcer, or non-specific colon inflammation.

A patient who has gradually lost weight, but seemingly has no digestive problems, is often suffering from hyperthyroidism. A person of this condition usually has a lower body temperature.

If a patient has all of these symptoms but exhibit hypocortico-hypoadrenal functions, then pigmentation will occur.

A patient who is a senior and is overweight, but steadily loses weight, may have chronic diabetes.

Besides this, the patient may also suffer from a chronic infection which is contagious such as tuberculosis, parasites, and hepatitis. If a patient is not treated for any of these illnesses and is still thin, then he may have cancer.

Stomach/Abdominal Pain

Often upper abdominal pain is indicative of acute gastritis or another type of stomach problem. Pain in the upper right abdominal area could be due to a gall bladder problem, cholangitis, or gall stones.

General abdominal pain could be due to hepatitis, or even pneumonia. Right lower abdominal pain could be due to the appendix and/or intestinal problems. Pain in the left lower abdomen is due to microbial infection or colonitis. Pain in the left upper abdomen is due to pancreasitis.

Pain along the side of the body could be due to kidney stones or a related excretory problem. If the area around the navel hurts, it could be due to the presence of tapeworms, or intestinal chyme impaction, mostly in the small intestines.

If localized pain becomes spread throughout the entire abdominal area, this signals that the entire abdominal cavity has become infected.

If there is sudden pain in the stomach or duodenal area, it could be due to an open late stage ulcer in the area causing internal bleeding. This pain is generally felt most severely after eating. Similar pain can also be felt if there is a parasitic infection in the area.

How can one determine if abdominal pain is caused by the appendix? If one lays flat on her back, takes a deep breath, filling it to capacity then holding it in for 30-40 seconds and expelling it quickly, you may be able to feel an extreme pulling pain. This would signal acute appendicitis, requiring immediate medical attention.

Drinking or excessive exposure to cold can cause involuntary muscle spasms in the stomach or intestines, or even gastritis. Binging often results in acute gastritis or pancreasitis. Pain when the stomach is empty may result from duodenal ulceration or gastritis. If one experiences pain in the upper abdominal area upon eating greasy or fatty foods, this is caused by the pancreas or gall bladder. If one experiences pain upon urinating, it could be a bladder infection or gall stones.

Young people who have stomach pains generally get them from ulcers and appendicitis. Those over middle age should be especially careful of the possibility of tumor growth if there is chronic stomach pain.

Gall stones are most commonly found in middle-aged, overweight women. Symptoms includes sporadic pain lasting from a few minutes to a few hours. This is normally due to either urethral or gall stones, or impacted feces.

With acute pancreasitis, pain will worsen as time goes on. It is important to get this condition examined by a physician immediately.

Knife-sharp pains caused by ulcers can be explained by the fact that the stomach is naturally acidic, while bile is alkaline. Thus, when the food mixes together, the bile reacts with and ultimately neutralizes the acidic stomach conditions, causing pain if there are ulcers.

Slight, sporadic colon pain is a possible sign of colon cancer. If the patient is over 30 years in age and experiences this pain along with bloating and irregular bowel movements, then precautions should be taken toward the early detection and prevention of cancer.

If a patient feels pain with nausea and vomiting, it could be acute pancreasitis, with an infectional impact on the intestines.

Stomach pain with diarrhea is cholangitis; with blood in the stool is possible cholera or tumor presence. Pain in the area without bowel movements or flatulation could be due to the impaction of materials in the intestines.

Normally people have soft, supple and smooth stomachs but if suddenly there is a hardened area that hurts when touched, there is a problem and diet should be lowered.

Of the main organs, the lungs are the most important to maintain oxygen balance and if liver functions are bad, with its prime function being to detoxify others, the other organs will deteriorate also. The blood circulation will be problematic, causing swelling and hardened areas. When lung excretions are poor, the most affected areas are liver and the digestive system. At this time, a hardness in the stomach area will be felt. Tumor is possibly located in this area, with the prime area being 2 inches away from the belly button.

Another symptom we can look for are white spots on the torso area, these don't have any feelings or lesions. These circular or elliptical pea sized spots will show toxins in the body. Recently, we have found that 800 cancer patients, 74% had these spots on the torso. If patient is immediately cured, spots will disappear soon.

Headaches

Generally, people get headaches from colds, fevers, or nervousness. These usually amount to small, minor headaches that will relieve themselves after certain amount of time. However, some headaches are more extreme and require special attention.

Headaches centered on the forehead are caused by disease of the eyes, ears, nose, or throat. Those that are caused by the eyes will also affect the vision. Similarly, a condition of the nasal passage may cause pain in the forehead along with pressure and pain in the nasal area.

Pain on one side of the head could be due to an ear infection, nervous disorder, or migraine headache.

Those above 60 years of age often experience aches in the temple area. This is possibly due to artery inflammation in the area that can irritate and cause headaches.

Headaches on the top of the head are usually caused by neurasthenia and tension. Headaches spanning to the nape of the neck in the back of the head (the occiput) may be caused by high blood pressure or kidney problems, meningitis or seizures.

Headaches felt over the entire head may stem from meningitis, concussion, neurasthenia, or atherosclerosis. Vigorous head pain, such as that felt when experiencing a migraine headache, may be caused by meningitis or high blood pressure.

Middle/older-aged people with these types of headaches usually have other symptoms of stroke and need to be extra careful. Scientists find that patients who experience brain blood vessel hemorrhaging that lead to massive bleeding and death often have prior symptoms including sporadic sharp pains. Warning signs in middle- to older-aged people include acute headaches but not fevers, nausea, or vomiting, or headaches that are severe mainly in the morning.

Sometimes stroke can be triggered by any excessive exertion of the body, such as a forceful bowel movement or heavy drinking, in which can the patient experiences excruciating pain. Stroke can also be triggered by other stimulating experiences and activities. Should one experience headache while exerting oneself physically or mentally, she or he should lie down flat immediately. Do not simply take medicine, unless it has been previously prescribed or the pain is not severe. Do not massage intensively or shake the head in any way that could make the condition more severe. If nausea is also experienced, lean back against something but do not lie down completely in case of vomiting and choking. If there is intermediate pain but it is not unbearable, this could be indicative of a brain tumor or an inflammation of eye diseases. If a light headache is accompanied by dizziness, then the patient may have anemia.

Pain in the back of the head that is especially painful in the morning and eases as the day goes on is likely to be caused by high blood pressure.

If one experiences headaches approximately 3 hours after eating, it is possible that this patient may have hypoglycemia, especially if it is accompanied by dizziness and sporadic pains.

Patients with brain tumors and parasinus conditions are likely to experience pain in the morning hours mostly.

Diseases of the eyes that cause headaches usually occur in the afternoon or evening.

Headaches that are felt late at night that are caused by excessive pressure in the eye, even after amounts of rest, are likely to be caused by iris infection.

Sudden sharp pain could be due to hemorrhaging and the bursting of blood vessels.

If one or both sides of the head throbs with the pulse, and the pain lasts for hours or days, accompanied by nausea, vomiting, and fatigue, it could be a migraine headache. Women experience pain more than men.

When headaches occur with throbbing and pressure, dizziness and worsening with shaking is caused by high blood pressure.

Pain from within the head, causing the sensation of a heavy head, always starting from the same point and expanding with time, could be due to the presence of a brain tumor. This generally feels worst from late at night until dawn and worsens when certain positions are taken.

Pulsating pain that travels from the forehead to the eye area, that is very extreme and lasts between a few seconds and several minutes could be the warning symptoms of a seizure.

If the head is swollen with a throbbing pain and the patient experiences insomnia and excessive dreaming during sleep, dizziness and fatigue yet does not have any disease prognosis, this person may have what is called a functional headache.

Chest Pains

Chest pains could be caused by organ problems, fractures, inflammation, or chemical or physical stimulation. The exact cause can be better diagnosed according to the area of pain.

Angina pain is normally localized in the heart area, and can be felt both in front of and behind the rib cage. Pain may irradiate to the left arm and the elbow area.

Acute pulmonary diaphragm infection or lung infection usually causes chest pain on only one side of the body.

Some pain is caused by pinching of rib nerves, leading to irritation in the area.

Progressive muscle pains in the chest area are caused by myoplagia and other pains.

Chest pain that does not span the midlength of the chest area is generally due to herpes zoster. There could also be chest pain experienced in the case of esophageal or digestive cancer, and eating will be difficult.

If the pain sears like a knife wound or pinpricks, along with a soreness in the area, it could be due to acute esophagitis, or angina. Those with angina will also experience pressure in the area, and the suffered may not even be able to breathe.

Chest pain with fever is often indicative of a respiratory problem such as pneumonia or tuberculosis-related pulmonary diaphragm infection. Chest pains with coughs and phlegm with blood, along with a feverish condition, usually signals tuberculosis or a bronchial condition.

If the patient has difficulty swallowing and is rather thin, then it is possibly a case of esophageal cancer. If there is chest pain with difficulty breathing, this could be a warning sign of emphysema. If there is chest pain, lowered blood pressure, pallor of the complexion, the tendency to have cold sweats, cold feet and hands, even coma, could be due to heart attack.

If chest pain and fever is experienced along with fatigue and difficulty in breathing, it is due to an epicardium inflammation.

All of these symptoms, since they relate to probably serious conditions, should be checked immediately by a physician.

Itchiness

If the skin is itchy over a lengthy amount of time, one can normally see the area that is affected since it is inflamed and reddish. However, if the affected area is not visible, then the itching could be caused by a variety of problems including diabetes, jaundice, and thyroid disorders. This could also be caused by chronic kidney infections and urine toxemia. If the area around the female genitalia is itchy (in the vulva folds) and there is a lot of discharge, the woman may be suffering from trichomoniasis or a vaginal yeast infection. Itching around the anus is sometimes due to the presence of colon tumors. Diseases such as leukemia, esophageal cancer, and lung cancer cause the entire body to feel itchy.

Female Disorders

For women who tend to have irregular periods, or spotting in between periods, this could be due to an estrogen imbalance, or another type of hormonal imbalance.

If there is vaginal bleeding during menopause or prior to menstruation, or if there is spotting or irregular bleeding, or bleeding after intercourse along with waist pains, this could indicate the presence of an ovarian cyst. Women between the ages of 40-50 should be especially watchful of this.

If the nipples secrete a clear, sticky fluid, this could be a sign of breast adenocarcinoma. Nipples that secrete a yellowish fluid signify a mammary duct problem, but does not necessarily signal a cancerous condition. If the discharge is brownish or reddish in color, then this definitely needs to be medically examined immediately. as it may be cancer in its late stages. 75 percent of women who have these symptoms after menopause have carcinomas.

Women between the ages of 50 and 60 should be especially careful of abdominal pain, poor digestion, and abnormally fast weight loss, as it may point to ovarian cancer.

Sleep Patterns

1996 Nature Magazine article shows that we sleep best around midnight, if there is no light. If the light is always on, then the best time to sleep moves to between 4 and 5 am. Thus, sleeping in a darkened room allows for better rest and a healthier daily rhythm. While sleeping, it is best to avoid any light sources.

If one sleeps on their stomach, then it is due to a weak liver. If one sleeps curled up in fetal position, then it is a kidney problem. If one sleeps spreadeagle on her or his back with an open mouth, then it could be indicative of a lung or bronchial weakness. If one sleeps spreadeagle on her or his back without open mouth, it is a circulation/heart problem. If the body is turned to the left but the head faces upwards, it is a stomach and intestinal weakness.

Urine/Excretory Functions

Normal urine that is excreted should be light yellow since urine has a yellow-colored substituent. If more water is ingested, then the urine is even lighter in color. If left outside for longer, the urine becomes darker. Since the body's metabolism is about the same, urine should be about the same color everyday. In normal people, there should be trace amounts of protein in the urine. There should be no more than 5mg/100mL of urine. Any more protein than that could signal a kidney disease or inflammation, drug poisoning, or be due to high fevers.

Urine placed in a test tube and heated over a flame with a

drop of vinegar should become clear as it boils. However, if there is protein presence, then the test tube will be cloudy as the proteins come out of solution.

If a woman's urine is cloudy, and still so even upon heating, then this is indicative of a urinary tract infection.

Bowels

There is normally a certain regularity to bowel movements, whether they be daily or more frequently than that. If the rate of movement becomes variegated, and the patient suffers bouts of constipation as well as diarrhea, then this may be due to colon problems. If the patient has abdominal bleeding and or pain in the area, with gurgling noises in the region and left abdominal edema, it could be due to this. Patients with rectal inflammation or rectal cancer often feel like they never have a complete bowel movement.

Mucous-caused blemishes are due to impaction of feces in the folded villi layers of the small intestines. A sticky, mucosy layer of material gets stuck in these finger-like folds, and with time, it forms a sticky plaque that deters absorption of nutrients and causes disease from the toxic uptake. The required treatment for this condition is a fast, followed by use of Cymosi Fibre-Cleanse to clear out intestines. Once the body returns to normal, all that is needed is the upkeep of the system.

Why does everyone like natural foods?

Advanced civilizations will find that medicine is not as good as adjusting one's diet. One must know the characteristics of foods, such as whether they are acidic or basic, cold or hot. Generally speaking, all grains, nuts, fish and meat are acidic. All vegetables and fruits are alkaline.

Those that wish to maintain a lighter diet should eat food composed mainly of alkaline foods, including cereals and nuts. Lighter foods mean better foods for your health, including usually only vegetarian entrees with very few, selected animal products.

Alkaline foods generally make people calmer. Monks, therefore, are generally calmer than the general population. On the other hand, acidic food eaters are generally more active.

In today's society, food and air suffer from environmental contamination, and an excess of acidic food intake will cause our cells to become toxic. Body fluid and acid/base chemistry will not balance. Adult diseases come more and more with acid foods. For better health, it is best to east less animal products and acidic foods, and depend more on alkaline foods for detoxification and recovery of the body's acid-base balance.
Alkaline foods, in order or their basicity, include the following:

Spinach, syrup, celery, carrots, green beans, cabbage, broccoli, beets, squash, mushrooms, cauliflower, pineapple, avocado, raisins, dates, tangerines, strawberries, tomatoes, yams, grapefruit, apricot, lemons, oranges, peaches, bananas, scallions, grapes, pears, apples, and watermelon.

Acidic foods, also in order from greatest to least acidic, include:

clams, sausage, oatmeal, lobster, peanuts, soda crackers, spaghetti, peanut butter, chicken, crab, beef, turkey, wheat, lamb, pork, pecans, smoked meats, eggs, bread, dairy products, honey, shrimp, corn, sugar, oil, wine, coffee, and tea.

Occult Blood

50 percent of ulcer patients have occult blood due to internal bleeding. Especially after treating it for over 1 and ½ months, special care must be taken as it may be symptomatic of a tumor. Digestive tumors include esophageal, stomach, and intestinal tumors. 20 percent of patients with occult blood have colon cancer. 40 percent have progressive stomach cancer. 25 percent of esophageal cancer patients have occult blood. Trace amounts as low as 2-4mL of blood can be detected in the feces as occult blood. In these conditions one will sometimes concurrently detect a dark vertical line on the fingernails leading to a dark splotch (Fig. 2-f). This confirms the possibility of internal bleeding.

For people who cannot digest fats well, their feces may have small droplike white fat particles or pellets.

Breathing Patterns

Is one's breathing regular? If you can hold your breath after inhaling normally for approximately 30 seconds, you have good lung activity. Each inhalation should inflate your lung cavity (pleural cavity) by 6-9 cm. Researchers have shown that a healthy tidal capacity should be between 3500-4000mL for men and 3000-3500mL for women. Upon exercise, the maximum capacity may reach 5000mL. The older one gets, the less volume one can breathe. Every 10 years after adulthood is reached should see a lowering of tidal capacity by about 9-20 percent. Boston University Hospital conducted research on 5,200 people for 2 years, and found that those who exercise regularly maintain good lung capacity even after the age of 60. Among 70 year olds, those who did not regularly exercise had an average lowered lung capacity of 20.64%.

Body Temperature

Normal oral body temps are between 36.2 to 37.2 degrees C. There is typically a 1-1.2 degree fluctuation, so when the body temperature fluctuates to more than 37.3, or rectally 37.6, then this is a bad sign.

Temp changes are usually due to changes in metabolism, so when one is eating or exercising, the temperature increases. Oppositely, when one is hungry, the body temp lowers. Children generally have a higher temp than adults, and the rectal temp is usually .5 C higher than the oral temp.

Fevers are often related to symptoms of diseases:

If the patient has a fever along with phlegm and heart pain, then it related to a respiratory problem.

Fevers along with abdominal pain, nausea, and vomiting are due to digestive problems.

Fevers along with frequent urination and urine bladder pain indicate excretory problems.

Fevers along with lymph node swelling and pain in a localized area is due to an infection in the locality. If lymph nodes on the entire body are swollen, then it could indicate TB or blood diseases such as lymphoma.

If fevers are accompanied by headaches, vomiting, dizziness, and comas, it is due to a central nervous system infection. Meningitis or viral infection and brain infections can also cause this.

If fevers are accompanied by bruises beneath the skin, this is due to meningitis, or it is a blood disease or lymphoma.

If the liver area is swollen, it may be due to cholera, malaria, or acute parasitic diseases.

Fevers that last for 1-2 weeks are typical length fevers and can be caused by acute diseases such as chicken pox, measles, scarlet fever, an upper respiratory infection or the flu, food poisoning or sun poisoning.

Any fever lasting over 2 weeks is due to cholera for a long period, TB, toxemia, leukemia, cancer, and so on.

Coughing

Coughs that are due to diseases may be caused by many reasons.

Acute coughs may be caused by upper respiratory problems, bronchitis, pneumonia, or diaphragm inflammation. Chronic coughs may be due to chronic bronchitis, TB, emphysema, or lung cancer.

Generally, short, slight coughs are due to pneumonia, or pulmonary diaphragm inflammations. Loud, hoarse sounding coughs are due to acute laryngitis. Coughing spasms that are not reflex responses may be due to diphtheria, whooping cough, rubella, or asthma. Night or morning coughs may be due to chronic bronchitis. Coughing in the daytime may be due to trachea or lung infections, or bronchitis.

If the patient has a lot of thick phlegm, it could be due to bronchitis. Rusty-colored phlegm could be due to pneumonia.

Coughs with fever are due to flu, lung inflammation, or tuberculosis. If it is hard to breathe, the cough could be due to asthma or heart failure. If there is vomiting with the cough, it could be due to rubella and or chronic laryngitis. If the phlegm is bloody, then the cough may be due to acute bronchitis, or lung tuberculosis. If there is a lot of blood, then it may be due to later stages of tuberculosis or bronchial dilation. Coughing accompanied by severe weight loss is symptomatic of lung cancer.

Skin

If the skin is really pale, it may not necessarily indicate anemic conditions in a patient. In this case one should also check the gums and lips and the sclera of the eyes. Abnormalities in these areas, such as pallor or pain, better signal an anemic condition.

If there are white, bean-shaped spots that are clearly defined on the skin, and certain spots where there is loss of pigmentation, this may be due to the effects of aging, if experienced in older people. However, loss of pigmentation may be due to genetic inheritance if it is experienced in younger people and may not be anything to worry about.

If the skin and the eyes are both yellow in color, then the patient may have cholangitis or pancreasitis, or there may be gall stones present.

If the skin is reddish, then there is a heart, liver, or intestinal problem. If the skin is bluish, then there may be a lung problem. If the abdominal area has lots of blue lines, that signals a lowered amount of adreno-corticosteroid production. If the skin has black spots, this is even further indication of the problem.

If the skin is dark and rough, then the patient must watch for stomach cancer signals. Patients with stomach cancer often start with the darkening or roughening of the skin as one of the precursor symptoms, occurring mostly on the sides of the body, inner thigh, and around the naval. In certain instances the face and the palm will also be darkened.

As people age, their skin will naturally get brown or black spots. This is indicative of what is also going in inside one's body. This type of pigmentation is also occurring in the organs of one's body, and can cause atherosclerosis if accumulated in the blood vessels, or fibrocystic disease. When these pigments are accumulated in brain cells, they cause loss of memory and senility. Those who are at this point in their lives need to ascertain that they getting enough water, selenium compounds (such as those found in Asparagus Extract), Vitamins B and C, cysteine, and vitamin A. These can be found in foods such as yeast, citrus fruits, honey, seaweed, milk, beans, eggs, and liver.

Purple-colored spots on the skin signal a platelet deficiency. Skin or membranes that have blood spots or bruises that do not change colors upon touch could be caused by meningitis.

Bright patches that show up on different parts of the body like dermatitis could be a pancreas problem.

Moles that get larger and larger and become irregularly-shaped should be checked immediately in the case of a malignancy.

Taste

If the patient notices a bitter taste in the mouth, it could be due to acute inflammation of the liver, or cholangitis. This has to do with bile acid metabolism which causes a bitter taste in the mouth.

This biter taste is also associated to cancer. Cancer patients sometimes lose their sense of taste to sweets and are increasingly sensitive to bitter tastes. This is due to a decreased circulation in the tongue, and a changed saliva constituency, which results in a chronically bitter taste in the mouth.

If the face is red, with red eyes, a bad temper, and dry stool, this may indicate a gall/liver problem. The tongue may be red with a thin yellow coating. If the heart is bothersome, the urine a dark yellow or reddish, then this may be cholangitis. In this case it may be very effective and helpful to take Liver Chi. (See appendix A for more details.)

If the mouth chronically has a sweet taste, it may indicate digestive problems. These patients often also have teethmarks on the sides of their tongue that support this suspicion. Diabetes is a major cause of this type of sweetness in the mouth. There may be an overproduction of salivary amylase, or it may be due to pancreas, stomach problems.

If the mouth commonly tastes salty, this could be due to chronic laryngitis (kidney problems) or if your mouth has ulcers (oral ulcers.) If the mouth tastes salty, it is usually a kidney problem. People with this type of condition usually also are fatigued, with lower back and knee pain. They may have ringing in their ears, and dizziness. Cold sweats and night sweats, including nocturnal emissions, are common, as well as the need to go to the bathroom a lot, especially is the tongue is fat and there is no coating.

If the tongue tastes sour, the condition may be related to

gastritis, or duodenal ulcers. These people may feel nausea and bloating upon eating.

If the tongue has no taste at all, this is usually when the sickness first starts or is almost better. This is common in cases of intestinal inflammation or a variety of digestive tract diseases. Post-operative patients also feel this, as well as those that are malnourished, or lacking in zinc and vitamins.

If the mouth has a fruity, fragrant taste, then this is indicative of diabetes. This has also to do with one's age. The young are more sensitive to this than older people.

Phlegm

If phlegm is white, it could be caused by bronchitis or pneumonia, or an overgrowth of candidas yeast. The imbalance of yeast in the body is what causes yeast infections in genitalia and/or overall yeast infections throughout the body. The natural balance of the body's bacteria and yeast is hereby disrupted, allowing for an overgrowth of uncomfortable yeast, resulting in a yeast infection.

If phlegm is green-yellow, then this may be due to a secondary infection, a virus caused bacterial infection.

Green phlegm signals jaundice of pneumonia.

Red or brown-red phlegm signals blood in the phlegm.

If the phlegm is pink-colored, then it could be due to acute emphysema. Don't give people of this condition IV infusions too fast, because if so, water may accumulate in the lung and the phlegm will be pink. The patient will need immediate intensive care.

If the phlegm is rust-colored, then the patient most likely is in the more severe stages of pneumonia. The phlegm will usually be this color for 2-3 days, at which time it will turn yellow.

If phlegm is chocolate-covered, it could be due to amoeboid or protozoan infection, which may infect the liver to have pus. It may also affect the lung and trachea.

Grey or blackish phlegm may only be due to environmental problems.

Mucous

Clear, whitish mucus that is transparent could be due to an upper respiratory infection or early stage of pneumonia.

Yellowish chunks in the mucus signals a cold or bronchitis, or recovery from pneumonia.

Thin, watery mucus with air bubbles signals more extreme forms of secondary bronchial infection.

Very thick mucus with yellow or green in it means that the lung has pus, or tuberculosis or late stages of lung cancer with infection.

If the mucus has fresh blood, and a lot of fibrous blood sinews in it, then this could be tuberculosis, or laryngitis.

If the mucus contains bloody air bubbles, it could be due to emphysema.

Sweat

We normally produce 500-1000mL of sweat per day. 98-99% is water, and the rest is urea, uric acid, and other inorganic salts. The constituents of sweat are similar to those of urine. It can help control and adjust body temperature, body fluid, and excretion of bodily waste. It can also help maintain skin pH to avoid bacterial infection. Thus, not sweating in very hot weather is very bad for the body. Those that do not sweat often have diseases like psoriasis.

Night sweats that include weakness, cough, chest pain, and loss of appetite are symptoms of disorders such as tuberculosis.

Constant sweating can signal many disorders:
1)hyperthyroid conditions, including heart palpitations, etc.
2)septicemia, smelly sweat, cold sweats
3)hypoglycemia, dizziness, fatigue, hunger pangs
4)excessive medicine intake, heavy metal poisoning; agricultural pesticides contain a lot of phosphates: lead, mercury, arsenic all cause the tendency to sweat.
5)puberty-related conditions, during adolescence and hormonal imbalances.

Cold Sweats

When the nervous system is suddenly excited, cold sweats are sometimes triggered. This can in extreme cases be due to heart disease, or heart failure.

If only one side sweats, this may be symptomatic of pre-stroke conditions.

Yellow stains caused by sweating on clothing can indicate the excessive urea content in the sweat, but it may also indicate liver cirrhosis if it has a fishy smell to it.

Breath

If the breath smells like beer without drinking, it is a lymph node condition. If it smells like garlic but none has been ingested anytime soon, it could be due to phosphate pesticide poisoning. Breath that smells like fermented apples is caused by diabetes. Breath that often smells sour and foul can be indicative of digestive problems. Breath that smells like ammonia or urine could be due to kidney failure or renalitis.

Breath that has a moldy smell may be due to liver disease. If it smells like stool, it may be due to abdominal infections or constipation.

Gas

Excessive amounts of gas may be due to interdigestive

problems or digestive ulcers. It could also be due to liver, gall bladder or pancreas problems. It could be due to an overconsumption of foods such as beans, potatoes, eggs, or ingested air. 99 percent of gas has no smell at all. Gas consists of 80 percent nitrogen, 2-19 percent carbon dioxide, and methane, hydrogen, and oxygen.

Gas can also be due to late stages of digestive tumor, ruptured tumors and bacterial growth there.

Urine Quality

96-99 percent of urine is water. Everything else there is waste, uric acid or inositols. Normal adults should urinate a volume of between 1 and 2 liters per day. (1-1.5L for women; 1.5-2L for men.) Urine should be light yellow in color, clear, with little turbidity or cloudiness. There should be a grassy smell, as urine decomposes to ammonia.

If urine is colorless, it could be due to excessive water intake, diabetes, or chronic interstitial renalitis.

If urine is white and cloudy, it could contain pus which would indicate infection in the excretory regions. This could also be due to parasitic activity. In children this is sometimes normal as it can indicate the presence of sedimented salt. There is the need to drink more water to ease the condition.

Yellow, dark urine may be due to dietary intake, for instance, one high in carrots and other similarly pigmented vegetables. It could also be caused by liver diseases or gall problems, since bile is passed along the intestines and through the urine, and if the intestinal bile is clogged, there is increased bile in the urine. Hepatitis is also known to cause a darkening of color in the urine.

Blue-colored urine is symptomatic of cholera, where there is high blood calcium and vitamin D poisoning.

Black urine is often an acute hemolysis problem in the blood. This may be due to a serious malignancy or an extreme case of malaria. The serum has lots of free oxygen and hemoglobin, and the urine is often black due to this. The ingestion of dopamines for the treatment of Parkinson's disease also causes urine to be black.

Dark brown urine is most often due to acute renalitis, kidney infection and hepatitis. Also, burn patients may have brown-colored urine. However, very active people may typically have thick, saucy urine.

If the urine is reddish, it means that it contains red blood cells. The body maybe hemorrhaging, or it may be due to high blood pressure, edema, and urine protein. Glomerular inflammation and lupus patients may have this type of urine along with fevers. Patients with kidney stones may have blood in their urine, as do prostatitis patients and those that have suffered regional trauma.

Stool Quality

If stool is mostly watery with little form, it could be due to intestinal inflammation, or poison of some form. If the stool is loose, this could be due to chronic cholinitis or eating excessive fatty or greasy foods.

Stool that has a lot of mucus may be due to colitis. Stool that is dry and pellet-like may be due to constipation or tumors. If stool is thin and strip-like, than it may be related to colon cancer symptoms. Stool with blood and pus may be due to colon cancer, or colon/rectal cancer or cholera.

Air bubbles in the stool signal problems in the small intestine, while dry stool signals colon problems. If material is sticky, but there is no blood, then it is colon problem.

Water Retention/Edema

Anytime extreme or abnormal swelling occurs, a hospital examination should be done immediately. The swelling may not impede daily activities or cause discomfort. In this case, the description may be described to be functional edema, and treatment would call for minor salt intake regulation, and the possible use of diuretic agents. Asparagus Extract is an excellent diuretic agent for this purpose.

Males should beware especially for foot swelling while females should watch particularly for head edemas, which are respectively more dangerous for each group than the rest of the edemas. Prolonged swelling of the foot can indicate heart disease, while swelling in the head and upper body area indicates kidney disease. Both of these situations call for immediate action toward treatment and regulation of edema. Localized edema, with red flashes and pain, could signal edema in a small locality on the body. If the face, tongue, and lips have an elastic feel and are swollen, then this is indicative of an allergic reaction to allergens such as different foods, animal fur, pollen and dust, etc.

Water Retention/Edema

Anytime extreme or abnormal swelling occurs, a hospital examination should be done immediately. The swelling may not impede daily activities or cause discomfort. In this case, the description may be described to be functional edema, and treatment would call for minor salt intake regulation, and the possible use of diuretic agents. Asparagus Extract is an excellent diuretic agent for this purpose.

Males should beware especially for foot swelling while females should watch particularly for head edemas, which are respectively more dangerous for each group than the rest of the edemas. Prolonged swelling of the foot can indicate heart disease, while swelling in the head and upper body area indicates kidney disease. Both of these situations call for immediate action toward treatment and regulation of edema. Localized edema, with red flashes and pain, could signal edema in a small locality on the body. If the face, tongue, and lips have an elastic feel and are swollen, then this is indicative of an allergic reaction to allergens such as different foods, animal fur, pollen and dust, etc.

Cell membranes have a specific permeability to water that increases and/or decreases according to bodily regulatory mechanisms that balance osmotic pressure to the external and internal environments of the cell. If the cell become imbalanced, the cells may shrink or swell to dangerous levels. In the case of bloating, the three main reasons for this are:

1)heart problems
2)kidney problems
3)liver problems

Patients that have swelling problems may suffer from function water retention conditions, but these may not be dire.

Bloating can be due to several external reasons, such as standing for long periods of time, which would cause foot swelling, or high temperatures, which might cause general swelling. People that are overweight generally also have problems with water retention, mostly in the leg and foot.

25% of women experience bloating during or before their period, along with insomnia, cramps, and mood swings. Pregnancy in its later stages may also see an onset of water retention.

Older people who suffer water retention often have heart, liver and kidney problems. Taking medicines such as cortizones, contraceptives, and antiseptic drugs all cause water retention.

Water retention caused by the heart can be seen in the ankles or throughout the whole body if the condition is extreme.

Bloating caused by kidney problems is the most common reason for water retention in people. There is also pallor in the face, along with urine blood and protein presence.

Bloating caused by liver problems, especially liver cirrhosis, commonly start from the abdomen and work down to the feet. The spleen and liver become enlarged, and the liver function is poor. Malnutrition causes this type of bloating, such as that associated with TB, and anemia. Blood serum proteins and vitamin levels are low.

Hypothyroid conditions can also cause bloating. Sometimes the entire body may be affected, and the patient will feel weak, cold, with yellowish skin and constipation, slow movements, anemia, and irregular menstrual cycles in women.

Part IV

Summary of Diagnoses

The following is a summary of different diagnostic markers described in the past chapters used to pinpoint problems in each of the five main bodily systems. It is a combination of fingernail and tongue examining techniques, including the other examination techniques as well.

Lung Problems:

If the patient has pulmonary and/or respiratory problems, the area of the tongue just behind the tip will be red, with a thin, white coating. The front side of the tongue surface may be raised due to swelling or there may be detectable raised red points which are related to allergy, asthma, or bronchitis. The pulse felt will be faint. Other symptoms include fever, aversion to cold, coughs, and headaches, and calls for a reduction of heat and improvement of the respiration and oxygen levels, a problem that can be improved by taking Synergen and Vein Lite.

If the nails have a rolled appearance, with tips that curl upwards and a surface that resembles rough glass in its opacity and texture, then this is also indicative of respiratory problems such as emphysema.

If the colors of the different parts of the nails are reversed, with the lunulae being reddish while the rest of the nail is whitish, then the patient may have respiratory problems such as bronchitis.

Greenish or purplish colored nails signal a serious case of emphysema. along with various other respiratory disorders. Ridges along the nails also signal respiratory problems, and perhaps are indicative of kidney problems as well.

Lung problems can also be detected if the patient has a pale, whitish facial complexion.

Liver Problems:

Liver problems leave the tongue dark-red with bruised edges and a dark or grey coating, or dark branched veins unside. People with liver disorders tend to have bloating stomach, very dry mouths with a generally bitter taste. Other symptoms include heart problems and a general feeling of warm discomfort. Dizziness and confused thinking may also be present. Treatment calls for the adjustment of liver functions and detoxification (of such toxins as heavy metals, etc.) by use of Vein Lite and Liver Chi.

If the fingernail has a black circular or oval spot, which do not move with the nail growth, then this is indicative of liver problems, and even liver cancer. If there are dark ridges that appear on the fingernails, this may also be indicative of a liver problem.

People with liver problems often have a greenish, sickly facial complexion.

Heart and Circulation Problems:

Generally, problems of the heart can be detected by looking at the pinky nail has large lunule and tip of the tongue, which will appear thin and red, and sometimes elongated. The tip of the tongue may also have a white coating accompanied by a faint pulse. Heart and artery problems can also be indicated by a purple-red, stiff tongue with little to no overall coating and a mirror-like, dry look. The pulse may be faint, even when felt under some amount of pressure. Other symptoms include diagonal line (wrinkles) across the earlobe, fever, perspiration, thirst, dizziness, aversion to cold, coughs, confusion, joint pain and headaches. Black or red spots on underside of tongue are caused by toxins. This condition requires detoxification of bodily toxins (including heavy metals, etc.) and calls for a reduction of heat and improvement of respiration and oxygen levels, as circulation decreases with the effects. Vein Lite is an excellent product of choice for these symptoms, for its oral chelative properties and ability to increase blood circulation.

Short, wide, reddish nails signal cardiovascular problems including high blood pressure, atherosclerosis and the possibility of stroke or brain hemorrhage (Pic.2-d).

If the tops of the nails are wide while the bottoms of the nails are much narrower, this could be indicative of the possibility of stroke and other cardiovascular problems. Stroke is also possible if the lunulae are oversized and quite large.

If there are less than 8 lunulae on all the fingernails and /or dark protruding varicose veins underneath of the tongue, then there is a problem with poor circulation. Patients exhibiting problems of this sort should take Vein Lite to increase blood circulation and repair the lack of oxygen intracellularly. Patients suffering from heart problems tend to have a red face, be quick-tempered and are easily fatigued.

Spleen, Pancrease, Stomach and Intestinal Problems:

Teethmark on edge of the tongue is the major mark of spleen, pancrease and kidney problems. Problems of the spleen also can leave the tongue a purple-reddish color, with a thick, yellowish coating that has a greasy look. The pulse will be felt upon medium pressure, and the other symptoms include congestion, vomiting, heat, and a urinary condition where there is only concentrated, small amounts of urine. Treatment calls for use of a diuretic and the reduction of heat, effectively accomplished by taking Asparagus Extract. Digestron will also help in spleen function and overall digestion.

If the patient has stomach, pancrease or digestive problems, the tongue will be thick and yellow with a spiky coating, sometimes cracking and she or he will have an overall dry mouth. The pulse will be strong, and other symptoms may include fever, perspiration, chest congestion, wheezing, rash, and constipation. This problem calls for the reduction of heat and excretion of waste, by taking the herbal product Digestron. People with digestive problems, as described before, can also have what is known as a geographical tongue, where the coating is patchy (Pic. 6-b).

If the nail is flattened instead of being slightly curved in appearance, then this signals digestive problems such as chronic gastritis.

If the nail is blackish or yellowish in tone, then the patient may have a digestive problem. (This problem may not necessarily be simply a fungal infection.)

If the nail has a red, black or circular spot, then this is possibly indicative of chronic gastritis. The black line on the nail which moves with nail growth may indicate internal bleeding such as ulcers. If the cyst on the frenula of inside of upper lip indicates intestinal problems.

Patients with stomach and pancreas problems also tend to have yellowish complexions.

Kidney or Hormone Problems:

Poor kidney function cause the tongue to be light red and the coating thin and dry. The pulse felt will be faint, and the body and face will feel hot with a ruddy complexion. Other symptoms may include fatigue, and hot palms and feet. Treatment calls for improvement of the kidney function and cleansing of the blood, through use of Asparagus Extract and Vein Lite. Kidney is also related to hormonal balance. When tongue has red star-like spots, problems often indicate an imbalance in male, female or thyroids hormones. Chi Energy has been effectively used to rebalance the levels of hormones and their output and usage in the body.

Kidney problems will cause the face to have a blackish complexion. If the nails show two horizontal white lines going across the entire nail, then this is indicative of chronic kidney problems or low blood protein. Ridges, which can sometimes be blackish or colored, and white spots on the fingernail indicate kidney problems and hormonal problems (Pic. 3-a). If the nails are a greenish color, then if the patient is pregnant, the child may have serious problems, and perhaps be stillborn. If the nails are quite short naturally, but the color still normal, then the patient may be infertile.

With these general descriptions, one can be able to tell the physical conditions of many, including this one involving a 51-year-old man who had suffered tuberculosis as a child and emphysema a few years back due to over 30 years. His health had been steadily in decline until recently when he spent over three hours in an unventilated room spraying mold remover, after which he immediately fell very ill. His tongue showed (see Pic. 8b) a thick yellow-white mucous signaling lung (and kidney) problems current and prior, teethmarks on the side due to spleen and kidney problems, and redness at the tip due to heart problems. He began treatment with Asparagus Extract, Vein Lite, and Mineral Infrared Therapy on the chest and kidney areas, and within two months, he had recovered to the point that the tongue was much less yellowed or white, although the heart still showed some problems (Pic.8c).

Appendix A: Remedies

Vein Lite

Unique blend of Chinese herbs that has been proven by China and Japan's Health Departments to have the capacity to improve blood circulation and cellular oxygen levels. It helps cardiovascular conditions and has oral chelation effects to remove heavy metals from the system and detoxify the body. It also has the capacity to increase the brain's acetylcholine and acetylcholine esterase levels which have been shown to help slow the effects of senility by promoting the memory-building mechanisms in the brain. It has been shown to have better results than NGF, Nerve Growth Factor. It also has anti-oxidant effects which eliminate harmful free radicals in the system while increasing SOD (Superoxide Dismutase) levels.

Use of Vein Lite relieves symptoms such as darkened lips, cold hands and feet, numbness of the limbs, and a generally poor complexion by increasing the circulation a great deal. In radioactive isotope marking tests, Vein Lite proved itself as a significant promoter of glucose anabolism so that the brain could more effectively obtain nutrients to supply the body with energy. It was also shown to be good for dilation of blood vessels and thinning of blood viscosity.

In an experiment done to the test the effects of Vein Lite, rats were placed in two groups, A and B. Group A contained older rats both with and without brain damage, and Group B contained younger rats both with and without brain damage as well. Half of each randomly mixed group were given Vein Lite in appropriate doses for 30 days. All of the rats in both groups were then placed in a maze, and the results were that the rats who taken Vein Lite retained a higher level of memory in both brain damaged and non-brain damaged rats.

Vein Lite has been a top-selling item in the Japanese market for years, since its effects are excellent for working people who lead generally inactive and cramped lifestyles and thus suffer problems associated to busy urban life and its crowded, polluted environmental situation. But Vein Lite is excellent for people of any living situation, and works to improve your health and memory in a natural, beneficial way.

Vein Lite contains Rhizoma Chuanxiong, Flos Carthomi, Radix Paconiae Rubra, Radix Salviac Miltiorrhizae, Radix Aucklandiae, and Rhizoma Cyperi. It comes in the form of granular packs which can be taken in any liquid between meals, preferably in the mornings, anywhere between 1-3 bags daily. Vein Lite comes in boxes of 30 packs.

Asparagus Extract

Another immensely popular product is special concentrate prepared from the whole plant of Asparagus Officinalis Linn. Asparagus is an important luciferous vegetable well-known to have excellent diuretic capabilities. It began to show an outstanding therapeutic effect on many kinds of cancers two decades ago. When studied, Asparagus was shown to contain high levels of oligosaccharides and trace elements of selenium, an anti-oxidant. Both oligosaccharides and selenium have been studied for their anti-cancer activities. Oligosaccharides may be a potent immune modulator which has been shown through in vivo experimentation to augment T-cell activity and enhance immuno-pharmacological functions, while selenium is an important co-factor to many regulatory enzymes. Asparaginase, another component of Asparagus Extract, has been shown to help stop tumor cell growth.

Based on clinical studies done on 400 tumor patients carried out in more than 20 hospitals in China, Asparagus Extract can has been shown to restrain and prevent the metastasis of middle and well as late-stage tumor cells. It may also promote the growth and development of white blood cells so as to improve the body's immunity. It also cleanses the kidney and liver, and strengthens the spleen and the pancreas. In fact, doctors have effectively used Asparagus Extract on patients who suffer kidney dysfunction, and even kidney failure.

Asparagus Extract is made from the entire Asparagus plant, including the roots, and each granule pack contains the finest natural ingredients that are found in the plant itself: Asparagosides, Asparaginase, Asparamide, with histones, oligosaccharides, selenium, and lysine. Each granule pack contains the extract of a half pound of asparagus plant and root, so the entire box of 30 bags contains 15 pounds of asparagus! 1-2 granule bags can be taken daily, in liquids, for long-lasting results.

Chi Energy

This herbal invigorator is particularly effective in promoting energy that benefits the adrenal glands and kidneys. It contains Herba Epimedi, Radix Rehmannhia, Cistanchis Herba, and Rhizoma Picrorrhizae. Chi Energy serves to balance the Yin and Yang components of the body, connecting and smoothening all the meridian lines and strengthening overall bodily Chi. It nourishes bodily power by restoration of the astringent function. Chi Energy is considered the super-tonic for sexual longevity and is an excellent method to balance male and/or female hormones and restore a person's vital functions.

Chi Energy is generally used by people with kidney or hormonal problems and imbalances, and also comes in easy-to-use granule packs that can be taken with any fluid. Recommended usage is 1-2 packs daily, taken preferably in the morning.

Cymosi Fibre-Cleanse

Cymosi Fibre-Cleanse works to cleanse the intestines by removal of bodily wastes and harmful toxins, at the same time lowering blood sugar and lipid levels. It is especially beneficial to those suffering from chronic constipation and constipation associated to old age. Cymosi Fibre-Cleanse also works to improve diabetic symptoms, hemorrhoids (pile), and high blood lipid symptoms.

Cymosi Fibre-Cleanse consists of natural polysaccharide polymers. This material cannot be broken down by the enzymes produced by the body, and thus is indigestible as it travels through the digestive tract. Its structural formula consists of many hydroxide groups, making it able to form strong hydrogen bonds with through dipole-dipole interactions. The hydrogen bonds that are formed when it is immersed in water allow the material to be soluble when mixed with fluids, forming a gelatinous substance which has the capacity to expand to up to 100 times its original coarsely granular size. This substance, when mixed with chyme, forms a bulky, moist mass that travels into the large intestine and triggers peristaltic removal of waste upon entrance due to its expanded size.

The naturally found bacteria in the intestine produce enzymes which are unlike those made by the human body in that they are able to digest the polymers of Cymosi Fibre-Cleanse, breaking them down to non-toxic organic acids. These acids act on the nerve sensors of the internal membrane of the intestine, causing a reflex reaction that triggers peristalsis of the tract and hence further aiding excretion of waste.

Sufferers of constipation experience much discomfort, and chronic constipation can lead to many diseases. Use of laxatives to relieve constipation can cause chronic intestinitis (intestinal inflammation) and diarrhea, but use of Cymosi Fibre-Cleanse has been shown to be safe and expeditious, with little to no side effects. It is a water-soluble cellulose that will mix with fluids and expand into a bulky matter. Made from a special formula including wheat husks and mushrooms, it safely adjusts the balance of intestinal bacteria, triggering the body's natural mechanism of waste disposal. Use of Cymosi Fibre-Cleanse is excellent for the safe relief of constipation, greatly reducing the risks of rectal and colon cancer.

Cymosi Fibre-Cleanse has more of adhesive capacity than water, so it increases the stickiness and bulkiness of food, allowing a delayed entrance of the food into the small intestines. Diffusion time for nutrients is thus slower, so sugar is being absorbed at a slower rate. This process works to lower blood sugar by 14% its usual peak after meals. At the same time, urine C-peptide levels will be lowered considerably as well. Blood sugar usage rates will be the same, as the herb does not alter the rate of cell activity, so no hypoglycemic effects will occur.

Cymosi Fibre-Cleanse thus acts to reduce blood sugar levels and keep them steady, reduce the rate of absorption of sugar into the bloodstream, and increase affinity of insulin sensitivity to target organs. It works to lower cholesterol levels of those who have high blood lipid problems by 20%, and triglyceride levels by 38%. High density lipid levels increase by 10%, but all these effects are not seen in normal individuals, so there are no counter-effects if taken by a non-diabetic.

Made with *pure* polysaccharide extracts from maitake, and the very special herbs bariey and rhizoma fagopyri cymosi, this unique product can successfully improve digestive function and treat bowel irregularity, removing excess bile and mucus. Cymosi Fibre-Cleanse can cleanse the intestines by removal of bodily waste, preventing gall stone formation, and lowering blood sugar levels. It balances the

Experiment 1:

#of patients: 47	avg. rate of b.m.	#(%)of those w/hard stool	#(%)of those w/dried stool	#(%)of those w/long strips	#(%)of those w/floating stool
before Fibre-Cleanse	3.33+1.16	39 (82.98%)	8 (17.02%)		
after Fibre-Cleanse	1.60+0.65*	5 (10.64%)	5 (10.64%)	35 (74.47%)	2 (4.26%)
post data	1.84+0.71	14 (29.79%)	17 (36.17%)	16 (34.04%)	

*P<0.001

Experiment 2:

		after Fibre-Cleanse		post-data	
	before Fibre-Cleanse	reduction	complete alleviation	reduction	complete alleviation
pressure	35	7 (20%)	19 (54.29%)	12 (34.29%)	13 (37.14%)
pain	13	1 (7.69%)	9 (69.23%)	3 (23.08%)	5 (38.46%)
appetite	12		9 (75%)	2 (16.67%)	6 (50%)
nausea	6		5 (83.33%)		3 (50%)

In another experiment, patients were tested with cholesterol levels of over 230 and triglycerides levels of over 16mg/dL. They were tested before and after a course of 6 weeks, taking two pills before each meal.

Results from the experiment are as follows:

	cholesterol (mg/dL)	TG (mg/dL)	HDL (mg/dL)	LDL (mg/dL)
before F.C.	242.89+49.86	298.02+25.42	41.67+9.11	148.12+46.18
after F.C.	13.41+37.67	186.91+133.16	48.02+15.06	135.60+34.54
P	<0.001	<0.01	<0.001	<0.05

	glucose (mg/dL)	SGPT
before F.C.	106.91+17.76	29.86+9.12
after F.C.	92.47+14.16	22.20+6.85
P	<0.001	<0.001

Fibre-Cleanse use has also shown itself effective in controlling sy,ptoms of atherosclerosis, while adjusting HDL and creatonin levels.

	TC/HDL chol. ratio*	HDL/TC ratio	LDL/HDL
before Fibre-Cleanse	5.091+1.75	0.17+0.04	3.68+1.13
after Fibre-Cleanse	3.77+1.15	0.22+0.06	2.93+0.87
P	<0.001	<0.001	<0.001

*a total cholesterol/high density lipid ratio of <3.5 is desirable.

	BUN (mg/dL)	Cr (mg/dL)
before Fibre-Cleanse	14.44+2.66	1.22+0.23
after Fibre-Cleanse	18.68+3.75	1.67+0.33
P	<0.001	<0.001

intestinal pH and bacterial amounts. Its botanical ingredients work powerfully to relieve acute and chronic constipation and its associated bloating and discomfort, reducing hemorrhoid flare-ups and anal fissures. beneficial to those suffering from elderly conditions such as lowered digestive rates.

Cymosi Fibre-Cleanse's herbal mixture is gentle enough for children to take. Its recommended usage is 2-4caps daily, taken a half hour before breakfast with plenty of liquids.

Whole Skin: Scar-Free Skin Care Ointment

Reported on by Newsweek magazine in 1990 as a medical and herbal innovation, Whole Skin works quickly and efficiently to heal and prevent scarring of any open wound, including cuts, scrapes, burns, and even works toward healing the scars of old wounds. Whole Skin stops dehydration for all open wounds, ulcers and lacerations. It has the capacity to reduce pain and infections, lacerations, as well as relieve and prevent allergic reactions on the skin such as eczema, shingles, and psoriasis symptoms, and other skin disorders. It stops the progressive necrosis of the burn tissue and heals wounds without scarring, reducing keloids. Its contents promote circulation by preventing blood stasis and clearing away toxic materials, removing dead, putrid tissue and promoting growth of new tissue.

Whole Skin has been used with fast, remarkably effective results by the Chinese Medical Burns Association, and is used with acclaim in several other countries as well.

Newsweek touts its ability to "not only ease the pain of burn injuries...but speed healing, reduce scarring and drastically cut the cost of saving lives." It contains natural products that are great for the skin such as sesame seed oil, dioscorea, bee propylis, and amurente.

Liver Chi

This product was #1 among the top-ten best-selling medicines in Japan for years, and its formula was featured in 1995 editions of the Wall Street Journal and the Washington Post.

Liver Chi is used by patients with chronic hepatitis, liver and stomach abnormalities which cause upper abdominal pain and vomiting, sour stomach, fatigue, a bitter taste in the mouth, and a reduced appetite due to a seemingly smaller stomach capacity. Liver Chi works by inhibiting viral replication, adjusting immunity to fight against viral infection, and preventing intra-cellular hepatitis viral outbreaks. The product is very mild and gives no negative side effects. It is highly recommended for those with poor immune systems, chronic hepatitis, liver fibrosis, fatty livers, and liver cirrhosis. It works to reduce liver enzymes, increasing liver cells' reproductivity, and has been shown to have a promote a recovery rate of 75% of chronic hepatitis sufferers.

The liver normally contains approximately 5% fat. In malnutrition, chronic infections of the liver and liver poisoning, e.g. from chronic alcoholism, chronic ulcers, cholangitis, tuberculosis, diabetes, serious anemia or tumor cachexia, the fat content increases in the liver, resulting in fatty liver. Fatty liver is reversible, however, and can be normalized after reasonable treatment. Liver Chi proves itself beneficial in experiments done in vitro, increasing T-helper cell activity and antibody action. This can directly stimulate phagocyte action and the peripheral mononucleoid production of interferons. It works to lower liver enzyme SGPT levels to normal in patients with hepatitis, as well as convert Hepatitis B surface antigen and core antigen from positive to negative, thus increasing hepatitis B core antigen antibody levels.

Mice which had alcohol-induced fatty livers due to high levels of alcohol in their diets were given 500mg of Liver Chi. Results from later examination showed not only reduction of fatty liver, but also a return to normal levels of lipid peroxidase in the liver cells. Also, tyrosine transferase enzyme levels actually increased proportionally to the amount of medicine taken.

Increased antibody production has been discovered upon consumption of Liver Chi both in the cases of experiments done in viro and in vitro, and in both cases there is also evidence of induced interferon production. Liver Chi proves itself beneficial to liver cell protection as well as liver cell membrane function. In vitro lympha cells activate and increase antibody action, activating phagocytosis and increasing T-helper cell activity. This can directly stimulate phagocytes, and the peripheral mononucleoid cell production of interferon. Tests show production amounts and rates to be stable in low levels in cultures, proving that Liver Chi is good for liver treatment.

Liver Chi is made with Chinese herbal extracts of Radix Bupleuri, Rhizoma Pinelliae, Radix Scutellariae, Radix Ginseng, and also includes methionine, bitatrate choline and aqueous vitamin B12. It is effective in reducing cholesterol levels while improving liver functions with no side effects. It now comes in both granular as well as capsule form, and can thus be purchased in boxes or bottles.

Digestron

This product has been shown to be excellent for stomach and digestive problems. Its special herbal ingredients allow it to reduces stomach and intestinal spasms while benefitting proper digestion and reducing excess gas. It also helps the smooth muscles contractions of small intestines, functions as an anti-histamine and an endorphin, and has anti-adrenocortico functions. The product not only works to improve stomach and pancreas function, but also has the capacity to relieve pain and lower blood pressure by dilating peripheral blood vessels. Also fights trichomoniasis and bacillus infection.

The ingredients that make up Digestron include Piper Longum, Aucklandiae lappa Dene, Cortex Cinnamomi and Rhizoma Alpiniae Officinalis.

Diabend

Diabend is designed to efficiently stimulate the secretion of insulin, and remove and prevent the binding of protein to insulin, thus allowing insulin to function uninhibitedly. Diabend is highly recommended for patients with type II late onset diabetes, as it adjusts and stabilizes sugar levels and usage rates in the system.

Diabend contains extracts of Allium satium, Radix scutellariae, Cratargus pinnatifida, Alisma plantagoaquatica, Lonicerae flos, Schizandra phinensis, and Ginseng, a unique herbal mixture that produces excellent results.

In China, 68.2% of 195 type II diabetes patients are reported to have good results upon taking Diabend for 3-6 months, blood and urine sugar, triglycerides and cholesterol were reduced. Doctors all over the world, and especially in the United States, have been using this newly developed formula with success. Diabend has the capacity to help produce saliva, quench thirst, alleviate mental uneasiness, and normalize blood sugar levels while nourishing the pancreas and maintaining a healthy appetite to help people suffering from diabetic symptoms. Diabend comes in capsule form, and patients are advised to take 3-4 capsules twice daily.

Myomin

Myoma is the most commonly seen abnormal growth on the female genitalia, and is also the most frequently seen tumors in the entire body. It results from the unhindered growth of smooth muscle on the uterus, and has the greatest occurrence between middle-age and menopause. Symptoms are irregular but include bleeding, abdominal pain, lumpiness in the abdomen, increased and thickened discharge, infertility, pressure felt in the lower abdomen, and affected heart function. Traditional western medicines have used factors such as age, various symptoms, size of growth, etc., to determine the best way to control the myoma, whether it be by surgical or non-surgical methods. Male hormones are usually used in the treatment of myoma, since they can antagonize the female hormonal reaction that triggers uterine bleeding and extend the menstrual cycle, controlling myoma growth. But side effects include of this type of treatment include liver dysfunction and imbalancing of hormones. Surgery, which may sometimes be necessary to sufficiently reduce the threat of malignancy, is an option that comes with many emotional complications as well as health risks.

The development of Myomin as a Chinese herbal treatment has been clinically shown to reduce myoma symptoms and significantly reduce the size and rate of growth. This amazing mixture has also been shown to help prevent ectopic pregnancy, adjust irregular menstrual cycles, prevent post-operative adhesion of organs, and now has been found to work on other tumors as well, showing an 88% general effectiveness rate.

Myomin works best on tumors no larger than 2-3 cm in each dimension. It increases circulation in the area and helps dissolve clots, detoxifying the system and mitigating fever. It is excellent for alleviation of enlarged livers and spleens and cirrhosis. Myomin has also been shown to be effective in the improvement osteoporosis and kidney problems. It contains: Fructus Psoralea, Poris Cocos, codonopsos pilosula, atractylodes macrocephala, crataegas oxyacantha.

Germanium-132

Germanium has been recently hailed as a regulator of the body's homeostasis and a normalizer of functions. It has proven anti-cancer value, especially against tumor growth and metastasis as well as the pain of advanced cancer. It helps to increase mental capacity, relieve sleeping disorders, eliminate toxic poisons, correct frequent urination, reduce allergic reactions, normalize and restore blood pressure, relieve pain and bring enriched oxygen supply into the blood cells. It has been used for hepatitis, diverticulitus, impaired amino response, chemotherapy problems, rheumatoid arthritis, external skin problems such as warts, acne, corns, and eczema.

Among findings from studies done on Germanium in animal and clinical tests was that the production of gamma-interferon (a major "biological response modifier" normally produced by the immune cells themselves) was boosted in animals and healthy human volunteers. On the other hand, it normalized antibody production in cases of delayed hypersensitivity/ "allergy" by having a damping effect.

Both in healthy human volunteers and in patients with cancer and rheumatoid arthritis, Germanium-132 normalized T and B lymphocyte function, Natural Killer (NK) cell proliferation, antibody-dependent cellular cytotoxicity and numbers of antibody-forming cells, all of which effects could stem from its ability to stimulate interferon production and act as a semi-conductor to clean out foreign materials in the body.

Maitake

Maitake, whose literal meaning is "Dancing Mushroom," is known to function as a potent resource to balance altered body systems back to normal. Recent studies done on maitake (Grifola Frondosa) have confirmed that it is more effective than any of the medicinal mushrooms previously studied in terms of anti-tumor activities as well as enhancement of the immune system. Researchers have said that Maitake contains unique compounds of high molecular weight and polysaccharides such as beta-glucan which makes it superior to other medicinal mushrooms including Shitake and Reishi.

The maitake mushroom is native to China and northeast Japan and has been prized in Japanese herbology for centuries as a method to strengthen the body and improve overall health. The compounds contained in maitake have the capacity to not only stimulate immune function, but also inhibit tumor growth. Recent studies have shown that maitake is also good for HIV/AIDS patients, as it may help prevent the destruction of T-helper cells by HIV. Some doctors even consider maitake to be excellent for inhibition of tumor metastasis, as shown in clinical reports which show results for breast cancer, pulmonary cancer, liver cancer, prostate cancer, and brain tumors.

Lily Hair Tonic

This herbal tonic is specially formulated to treat and prevent hair loss in both men and women. It is very effective toward increasing blood circulation, eliminating blood stasis, and stimulating receptor cells in hair follicles. It has the capacity to maintain a permanently conducive growth condition on the scalp, and has been shown to be excellent for such conditions as alopecia and dandruff.

One should use Lily Hair Tonic as a salve, pouring a few drops into the palm of the hand and massaging it into the affected area of the scalp after shampooing. It is also suggested that one places a moist, hot cloth over the area after applying the tonic as this will allow for pores to open up and better absorb the herbal ingredients. This should be done very consistently at least once a day if there are to be good results seen. Lily Hair Tonic contains: Cortex Phellodendri, Radix Sophorae Flavescentis, Ructus Chidii, and Rhizoma Atracylodis.

Slender All

Slender functions to speed metabolism and adjust fat catabolism for a naturally slimmer physique. It works to remove the excess ADP in the metabolic pathways that block the process of fat catabolism, expediting the burning process of fat. Thus, Slender All should be taken before exercising for best results.

Slender All contains Allium satium, Crataefus pinnatifida, Raphamus sativus, Rheum palmatum, Zingiver officinale, and Schizandra Chinensis.

Happy Skin Tonic

This all-natural cleanser functions as a mild yet highly effective disinfectant that diminishes genital and vaginal inflammation due to bacteria, fungi, or trichomonal infections and shows a direct killing-effect on Type 2 herpes and gonococcus. It has excellent clinical efficacy on gonorrhea and is especially effective on bacterial vaginitis. It is also good for preventing perennial wound infections and is specifically developed to prevent genital organ diseases as well as pruritus, eczema and cruristinea.

Happy Skin Tonic can be used as a lotion or liquid for external use in the genital area as an agent to eliminate undesirable odors, making one feel fresh and comfortable. It can be used before and/or after intercourse to promote sanitation, or after child-birth in order to prevent disease or infection.

Clinical studies show that Happy Skin Tonic has an effectivity rate of 95% in treating various vaginitis and pruritus vulvae. The extent of its effect on eczema, tinea, dermatitis, and persistent itching has an effective rate of 87%. Happy Skin Tonic can also produce excellent results in the treatment of tinea, eczema, scabies, dermatitis, and beriberi.

Besides genital infections and cleansing, Happy Skin Tonic can be used to relieve athlete's foot, nail fungus, and other external fungal and bacterial infections. It contains Cortex Phellodendri, Radix Sophorae Flavescentis, Ructus Chidii, and Rhizoma Atractylodis, and can be applied twice a day or as the patient sees fit.

Synergen

This brand new herbal product has been shown to be excellent for treating lung problems, one of the main ones being lung disease. The main symptoms of this disease include asthma and shortness of breath, coughing and blood in the pus. Patients will have edema throughout the entire body, and may have trouble urinating or suffer from constipation. Synergen is also especially good for seasonal asthma, and should be taken for this *before* the attacks arrive for best results.

Another problem that Synergen treats is simply poor lung functions. These patients will have coughs and asthmatic symptoms with a faint, low voice and fatigue throughout the body. The person's phlegm will be light-colored and thin, with a clear, mucusy feel. The face will appear pale and sallow, and the patient may be susceptible to colds, with excessive sweating and an aversion to cold conditions. Synergen is also good for patients who have dry coughs with little or no phlegm, or those with very sticky phlegm. For these people, the area around the lung may feel hot, and there may be a low degree fever felt, and excess of sweat. The tongue of this condition will be a red or purple-red color, with liver saliva and a weak pulse.

Synergen is made of a unique botanical mix of all-natural herbal ingredients, including Radix Scrophulariae, Radix Rehmanniae Praeparata, Fructus Psoraleae, Herba Epidemii, Semen Cuscutae, and Pericarpium Citri Reticulatae.

Saliva Ovulation Test Kit

A quick and accurate new way to determine the female ovulation period, this portable microscope can determine the body's most fertile periods safely and naturally using nothing but one drop of saliva. It is also really important for female hormonal control. One way to detect a hormonal imbalance is to follow the body's cycle as it travels through its fertility phases:

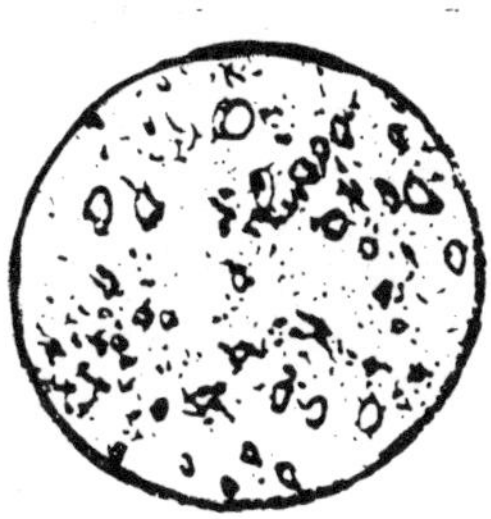

Infertile Period
98% accurate

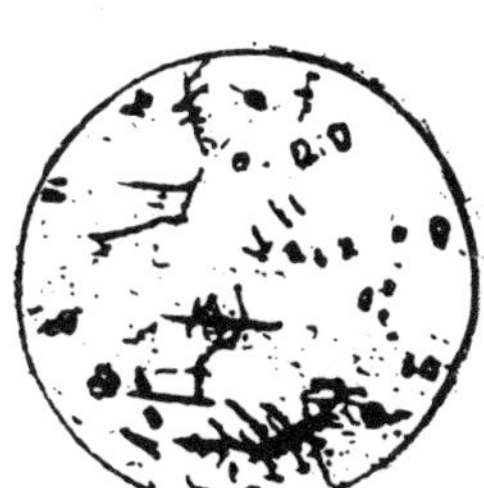

Transitional Period
94% accurate; 6% may be infertile

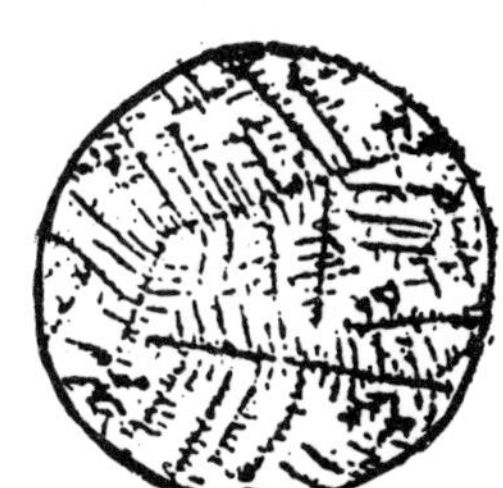

Fertile Period
>99% accurate

OVUSCOPE ACCURACY TEST FROM A CHINA HOSPITAL

In a November 25, 1995 report, the Ob/Gyn department in a hospital in China performed an ovulation test on 50 women. Their ages ranged from 18 to 42 years of age with an average age of 28. Their average menstruation lasted four to six days and their average menstrual cycle was between 28 and 31 days. None of the women were pregnant at the time of these tests.

The fifty women were tested by the female ovulation test called the Ovuscope and then by the normal, clinical way of examing their vagina's cervical fluid under a clinical microscope. All participants did not eat, drink, or smoke for two hours before the tests. The women applied their saliva on the inside glass of the microscopes and let it air dry.

	OVULATION STAGE	TRANSITIONAL STAGE	INFERTILE STAGE
CONTROL GROUP	6	21	23
TEST GROUP	6	20 *	21**
PERCENT ACCURATE	100%	95.2%	91.3%

* One found by Ovuscope is in her infertile period.
** Two found by Ovuscope are in their transitional period.

The Ovuscope has an average accuracy of 94% and is >99% accurate during a women's fertile period.

The Ovuscope has many advantages. Due to the change in the content of salts and hormones in a women's body, the Ovuscope is able to determine which stage of fertility she is currently in. This can be useful for women who are trying to get pregnant and for women who are using it not to get pregnant. It is quick, accurate and easy to use. Since it is the size of a women's lipstick, it is easy to conceal and carry on you.

Generally, the cycle spends 6-8 days in the infertile period, followed by 3-4 days in the transitional period, and then 1-2 days in the fertile period. However, if one notices that her cycle is irregular to the point of shifting constantly between the infertile and transitional period, then she has a hormonal imbalance.

The physiological changes that take place within the female body during each monthly cycle reflect themselves not only in the body's temperature, but also in the content of hormone and salt in the saliva. The tiny test microscope is easy to use and long-lasting. Simply unscrew the lens head, smear a small amount of saliva onto the inside glass with a toothpick, wait 5-7 minutes for the sample to dry, then screw the head back on and look into the lens while pressing the light button on the other side and adjusting the focus until the picture in clear. Fertile periods are seen as branch-like patterns on the lens, while infertile periods are seen as small dispersed bubbles throughout the lens. Transitional periods (when there is a chance for fertility) are seen as both bubbles and branches.

It is best to test saliva in the mornings, at least two hours after smoking, drinking or eating. Wipe lens clean after each use with wet cloth, but do not submerge microscope with water or alcohol.

Mineral Infared Therapy

The mineral infrared frequency device with portioned electromagnetic spectrum is an entirely new concept in medical technology. In essence, the device functions to give off proper bioenergy promote enzyme funciton and metabolism by activating trace elements in our body, regulate physiological deficiencies, diminish and heal inflammations, and relieve pains. In brief, the mineral frequency device creates electromagnetic waves within a certain range of the spectrum by translating the energy of the heating element to produce the electromagnetic waves. The waves enter the body as mineral infrared waves and increase organ functions. The thirty-three different trace elements in the mineral coated plate are related to the elements found in the human body, and have been found to yield therapeutic effects on the human body such as:

- the relief of muscular aches and pains caused by arthritic and soft tissue injuries
- the alleviation of inflammation and edema from soft tissue injuries
- the assistance in the healing of skin disorders
- the balancing of the nervous system
- the promotion of healing effects on internal organs, and
- the treatment of bone fractures

The device is thus excellent for treatment of the mineral insemination problems discussed in early chapters. These are but a few of the wonderful effects of mineral infrared therapy. More about the theory and application of this remarkable device can be found in my last book, *Dr. Chi's Guide to Health with Mineral Frequency and Herbs*.

Appendix B: Herbs

The following is a list of herbs, many of which are included in Chi's Enterprise herbal products, and their uses:

Aucklandia lappa Dene
Reduces spasms, good for the central nervous system. Good for the bronchioles and helps the smooth muscles contractions of small intestines. Functions as an anti-histamine and an endorphin, has anti-adrenocortico functions. Relieves pain and lowers blood pressure by dilating peripheral blood vessels. Also fights trichomoniasis and bacillus infection.

Cacumen Biotae
Functions to detoxify blood, stops bleeding. Reduces phlegm in the mouth and stops coughs.

Cortex Cinnamomi
Relieves pain, increases warmth, nourishes the spleen.

Cortex Phellodendri
Reduces fever, detoxifies the system, especially in post-partum conditions. Acts as a diuretic.

Endothelium Corneum Gigeriae Galli
Improves digestive function helps correct impotence. Helps spleen and stomach.

Eupolyphaga Seu Steleophaga
Detoxifies the bodily system, improves circulation and helps in the healing of bone injuries.

Flos Carthomi
This herb functions to stop blood stasis.

Flos Lonicerae
Reduces heat, detoxifies the system. Helps arthritis, is good for the meridian points and helps circulation.

Flos Lonicerae
Reduces fever, detoxifies the bodily systems.

Fructus Citri Sarcodactylis
Cleanses the liver, balances the bodily systems, detoxifies.

Fructus Psoraleae
Good for spleen and kidney potency. Also helps lung and blood vessel flux. Protects and increases white blood cell count after radiation therapy-caused deficiency.

Fructus Psoraleae
Improves kidney and sex organ function. Helps urine bladder function.

Fructus Schisandrae
Nourishes the lung and kidney, makes more saliva and allows it to flow easily. Also functions to calm the nerves, and has been shown to be good for the heart. This herb can also alleviate diarrhea.

Fructus Cnidii
Anti-infection, good to fight against cold or arthritis. Also good for kidney and sexual functions.

Fructus Piperis Longi
Balances the bodily systems, relieves pain.

Herba Agastachis
Acts as a diuretic and a fever reducer. Helps stop vomiting and relieves tinea.

Herba Epimedii
Good for kidney function, impotence, bone and tendon repair. Stops coughs and asthma. Cuts down on bronchial spasms. Anti-asthma effects; can also relieve inflammation and pussing. Dilates blood vessels and reduces blood sugar amount. Normalizes pulmonary blood vessels and functioning.

Herba Houttuyniae
Detoxifies, reduces fevers, good for relieving urinary tract infections. Also helps to expel pus from the system.

Pericarpium Citri Reticulatae
Dissolves phlegm and stops coughing. Improves spleen function by stimulating respiratory tract mucus membranes for expulsion of dissolved phlegm. Rids of stomach gas.

Pollen Typhae
Stops bleeding and blood stasis. Acts as a diuretic.

Poria
Acts as a diuretic, helps the spleen. Also functions to promote relaxed sleep.

Radix Bupleuri
Reduces fever in the body. Also works to cleanse the liver,

and is good for digestion.

Radix Codonopsis Pilosulae
Balance the body's systems, improves saliva function, and nourishes the blood.

Radix Rehmanniae Praeparata
Excellent for prevention of heart problems and heart failure. Helps inflammation and inhibits pus excretion. Anti-inflammatory effects as well.

Radix Salviae Miltiorrhizae
Improves circulation, prevents and relieves blood stasis, reduces fever, stops pain.

Radix Scrophulariae
A medium dose of this herb can allow strengthening of the heart during contractions, and a decrease of oxygen usage in the heart muscles. It is good for fungal infections, and helps reverse the effect of reduction in cell platelets due to radiation treatment.

Radix Stemonae
Helps to improve lungs and respiratory function, stopping coughs. Stops bacteria and parasites.

Radix Vladimiriae
Relieves pain, and balances the bodily systems and meridian points.

Radix Angelicae Dahuricae
Improves circulation, reduces pain and swelling, expels pus.

Radix Polygoni Multiflori
Good for the kidneys and hair. Helps sperm and blood, detoxifies and is good for constipation.

Radix Paeoniae
Reduces fever and cleanses blood of toxins. Very good for increasing circulation and relieving pain.

Radix Rehmannia
Reduces fevers and heat, cleans blood, good for bodily fluid.

Radix Astragali seu Hebysari
Helps potency and energy, relieves external and internal sores, and functions in the regeneration of tissue. Also helps relieve edema and act as a diuretic.

Radix Aconiti Praeparata
Restores potency, warms the body, good for colds, relieves pain, and balances meridian points.

Radix Panacis Quinquefolii
Reduces fevers, good for the saliva and bodily fluid. Fights fatigue and weakness.

Rhizoma Coptidis
Reduces fever, acts as a diuretic, detoxifies the system.

Rhizoma Liguistici Chuanxiong
Improves circulation, relieves arthritis and pains.

Rhizoma Dioscorea
Restores and improves spleen and kidney function.

Rhizoma Zingiberis
Warms the body, good for the lungs, stops bleeding.

Rhizoma Cyperi
This herb cleanses the liver, stops the symptoms of menopause, and works to relieve pain.

Rhizoma Atractylodis
Helps digestive function, mostly in the spleen. Improves sweat gland function, good for arthritis and eyes.

Rhizoma Atractylodis Macrocephalae
Improves spleen function, acts as a diuretic, prevents excess sweating.

Rhizoma Alpiniae Officinarum
Nourishes spleen and stomach, anti-bacterial.

Rhizoma Alismatis
This herb is a known diuretic, and is good for cleansing the kidney, thus improving excretory function.

Semen Raphani
Helps the stomach and digestive tract, reduces the bloating sensation in the abdomen. Also detoxifies the bodily systems.

Semen Cuscutae
Helps kidney and sperm. Reduces blood pressure, increases strength in heart contractions.

Semen Cassiae
This herb has the capacity to cleanse the liver, thereby

brightening the eyes. It has also been known to correct bowel irregularity and act as a diuretic.

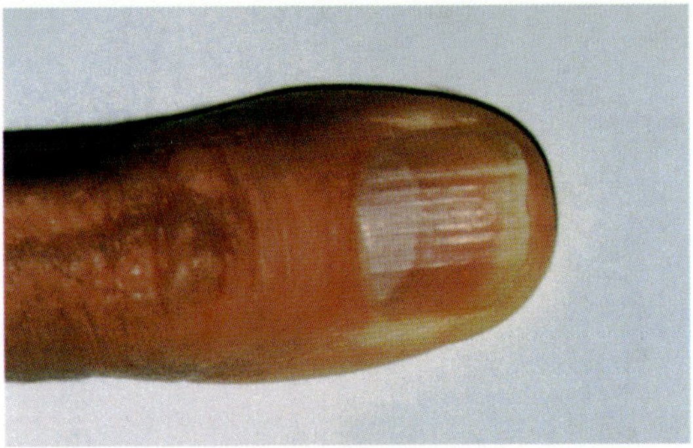

1 a

Thumbs have ridges:
Kidney.

Beads-on-a-string:
Arthritis, Osteoporosis.

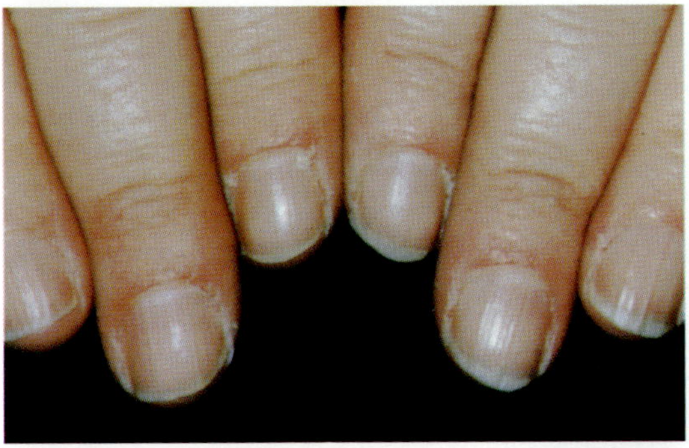

1b

Vertical ridges on every finger:
Respiratory problems.

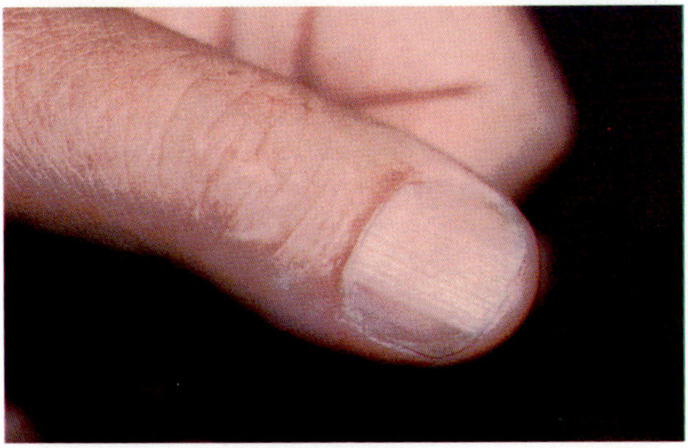

1c

Vertical ridges split:
Adrenals.

Very thin parallel lines:
Mineral insemination problems.

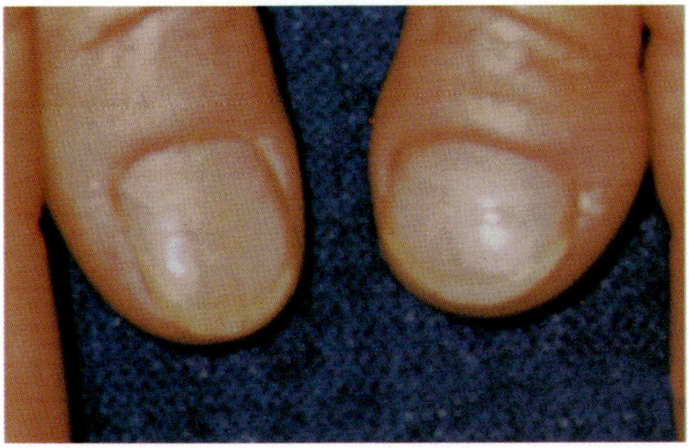

1d

Short, wide nails:
Heart condition.

Hazy boundaries between lunulae & flesh:
Hot / cold mix type.

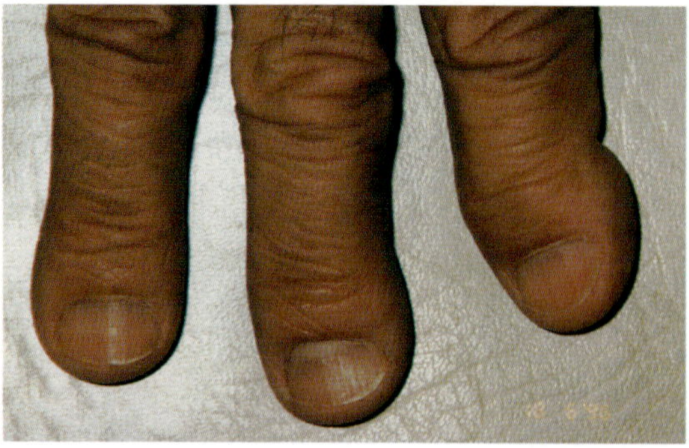

2a

Shot, wide nails, or fingertips:
Heart disease, poor circulation.

Spoon-shaped :
Anemia.

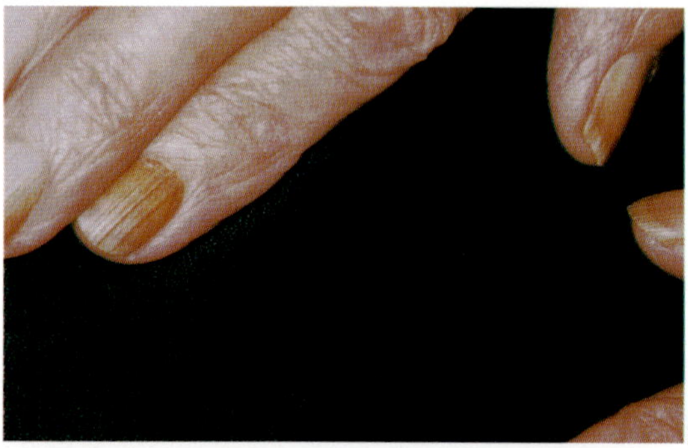

2b

Thumbs ridges:
Kidneys problems.

Others ridges:
Respiratory problems.

Yellow nails:
Digestion problems.

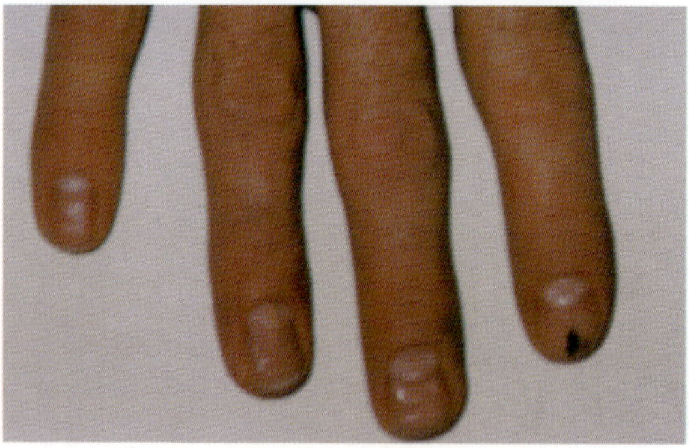

2c

Lunulae on pinky:
Heart condition.

Horizontal ridges:
A more serious case either because of cardiovasular or malnutrition.

Black spots:
Internal bleeding or digestion problems.

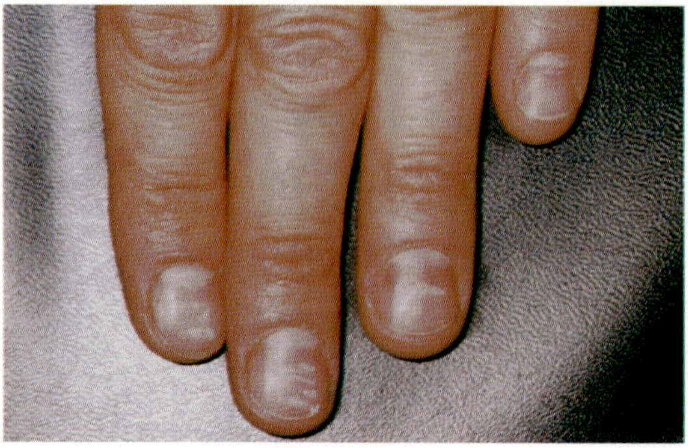

2d

White strips and spots:
Urine protein,
Kidney problems.

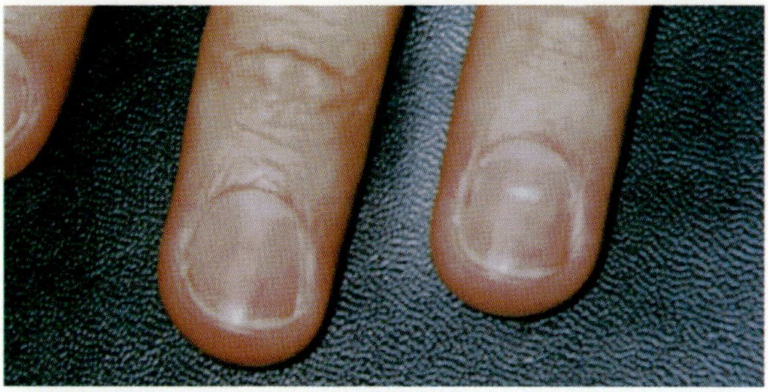

3a

White spots on nail:
Hormonal imbalance.

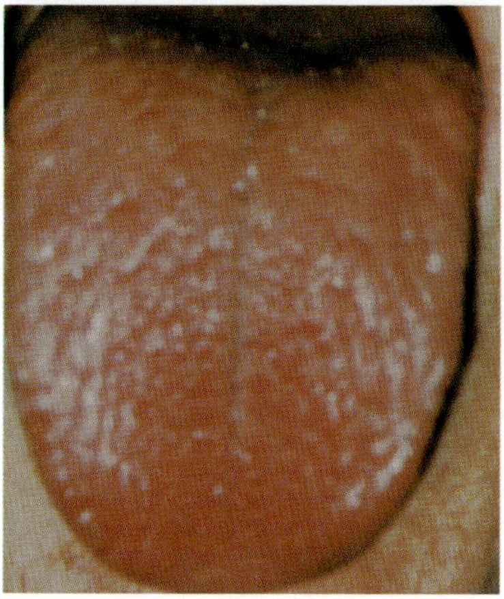

3b

No vitality:
No saliva; dry;
no energy;
poor digestion;
poor absorption.

Teethmarks:
Spleen pancreas problems, poor digestion, low immunity.

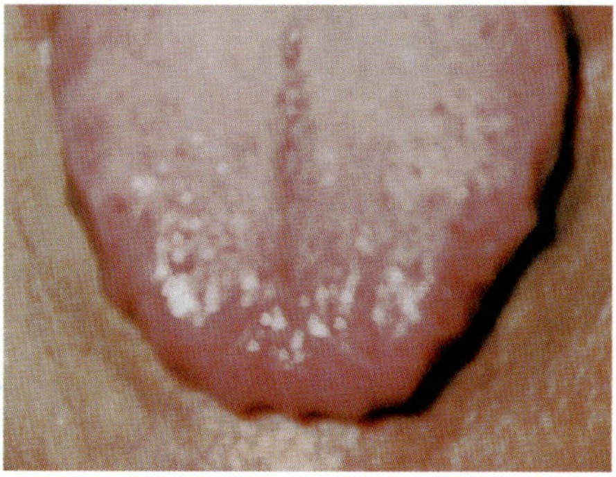

3c

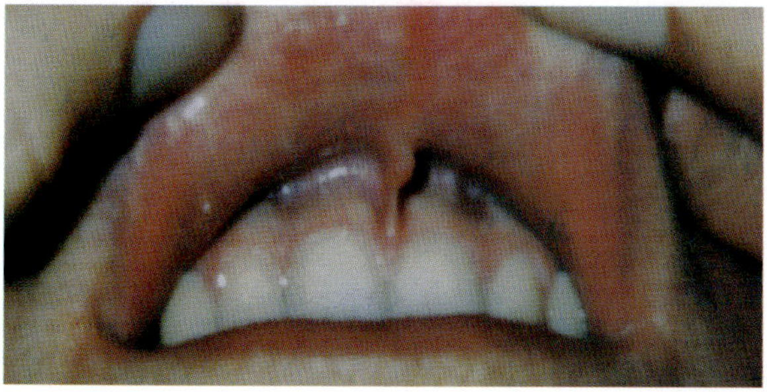

3d

Cyst on frenula (on top) secondary bile salts from liver bile accumulated on small intestines.

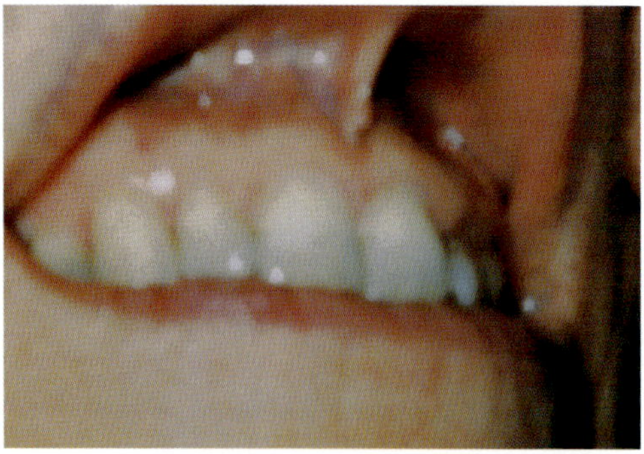

4a

Cyst on frenula (close to gum):
Affects large intestines.

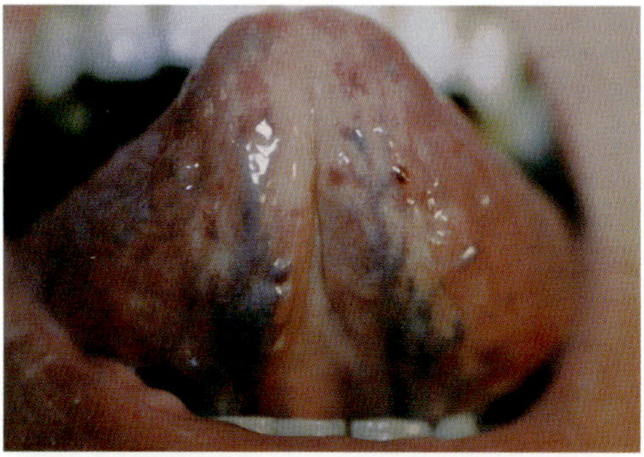

4b

Protruding Veins:
Poor circulation, if dark, then even more carbon dioxide present.

Red spots shown on the underside of the tongue:
Heavy metals accumulate.

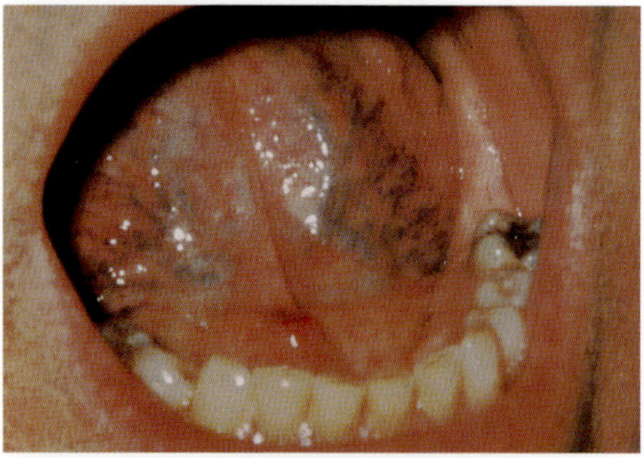

4c

Red/dark spots on botton of the tongue:
Heavy metal poisoning especially mercary from amalgam fillings.

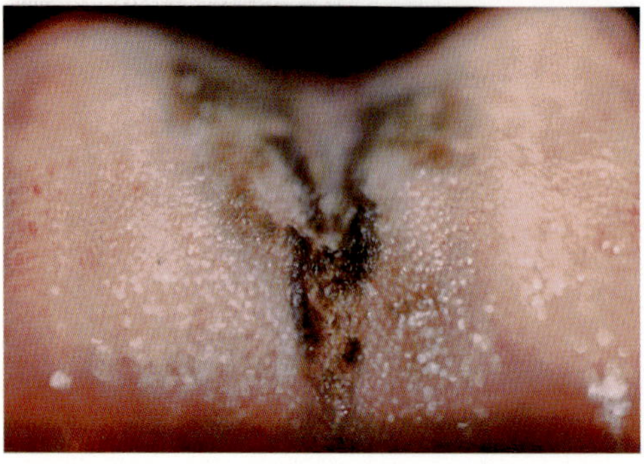

4d

Root of tongue turns from white to yellow to black; unable to be scraped off:
Serious Kidney problems.

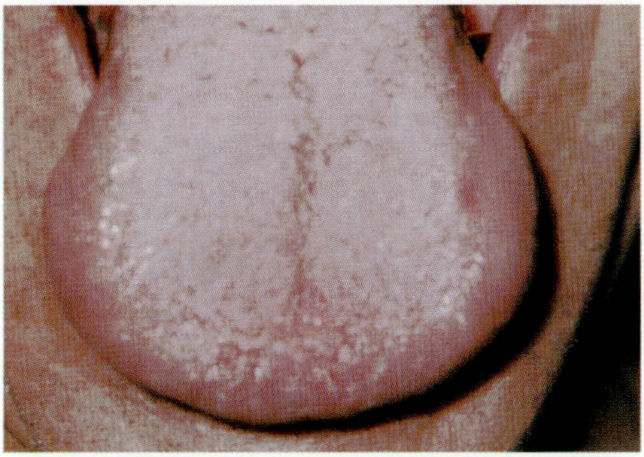
5a

Hammer-shaped tongue:
Hormone depletion, patient is over-sexed, kidney problems.

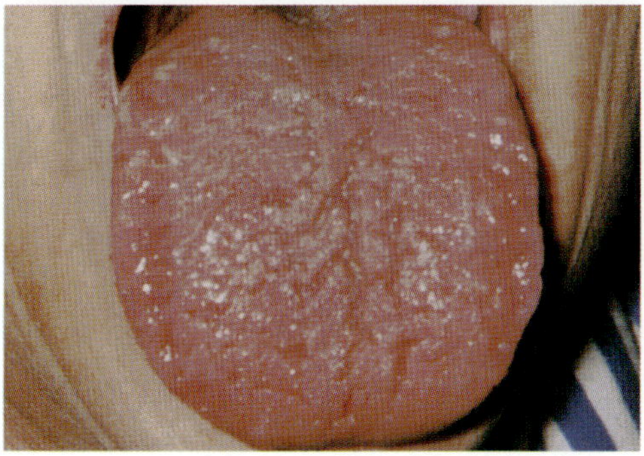
5b

Fissured tonque:
Poor digestion (espeical lambda shaped cracking) stomach, pancrease problems.

Marks on the side:
Signify problems in the spleen.

Yellow / brown coating in the back or root of the tongue:
Signals early kidney problems.

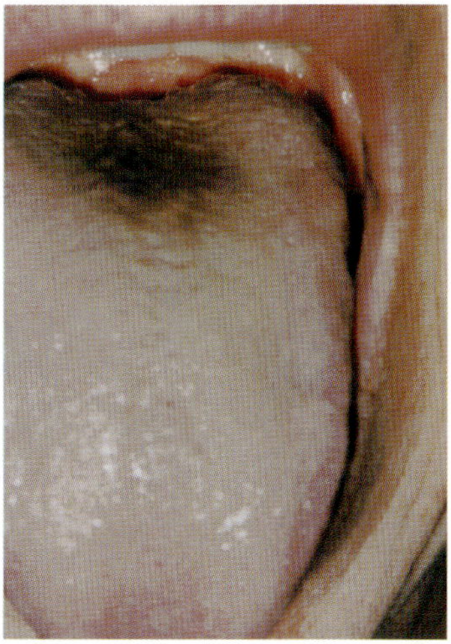
5c

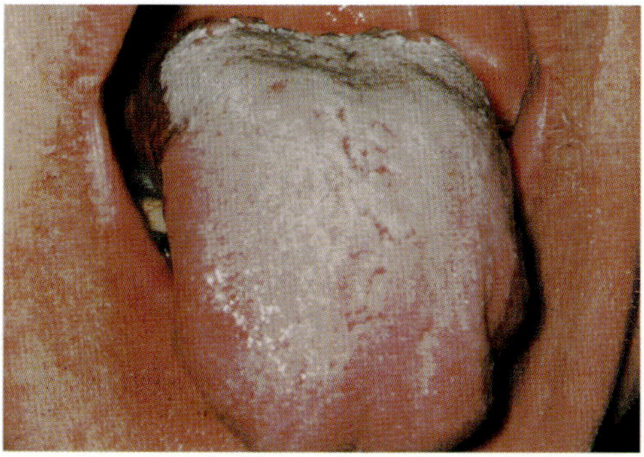
5d

White coating:
Respiratory problems.

White, greasy chunks:
Pneumonia.

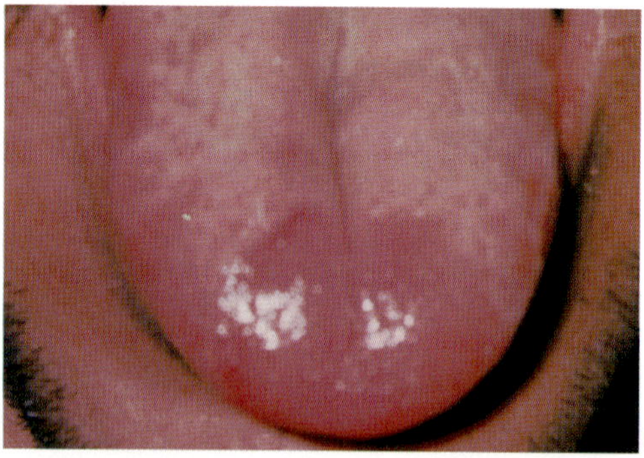

6a

Geographical, white-patchy tongue:
Could be due to allergies or sinus problems.

Red dots on side of the tongue:
Asthma.

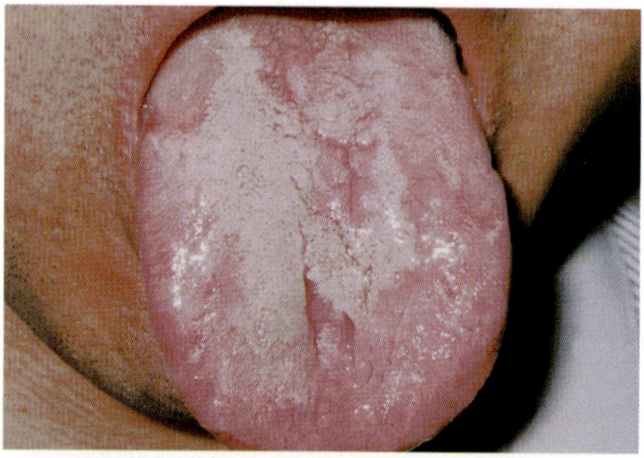

6b

Another case of geographical tongue, off-white coating, cracking, very patchy:
Poor digestion.

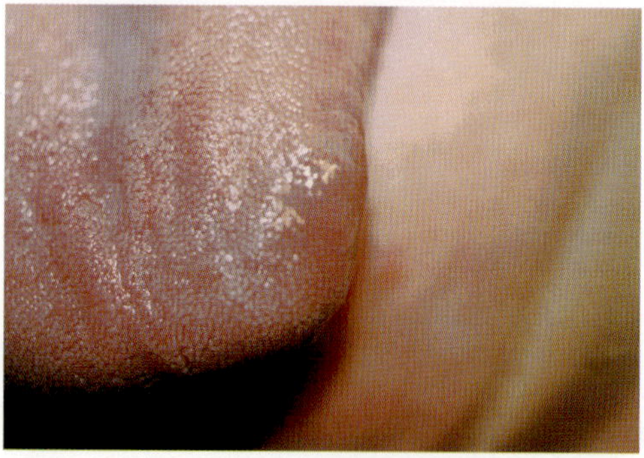

6c

White coating, side bulging:
Lung problems, asthma.

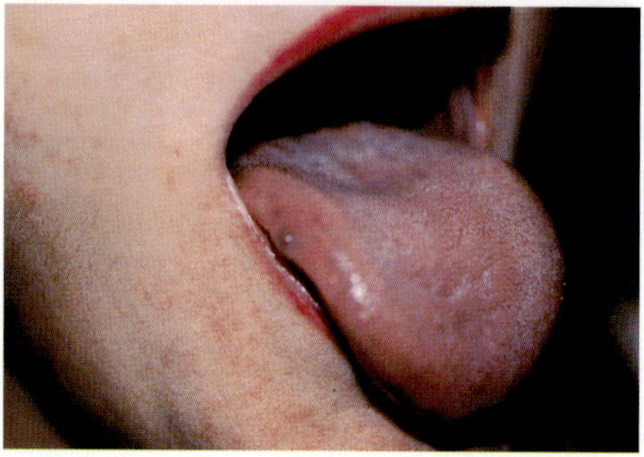

6d

Bruised spots or marks on the side of the tongue:
Liver and poor circulation.

On the right side:
May also be gall bladder problems.

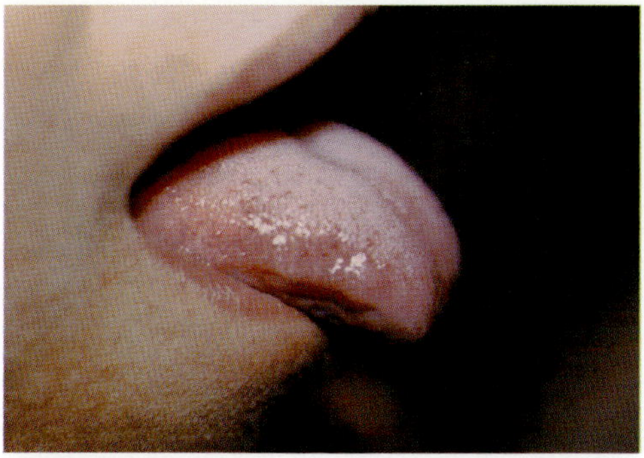

7a

Protrusion spots on the side of the tongue:
Poor liver function; could also be female menstrual problems.

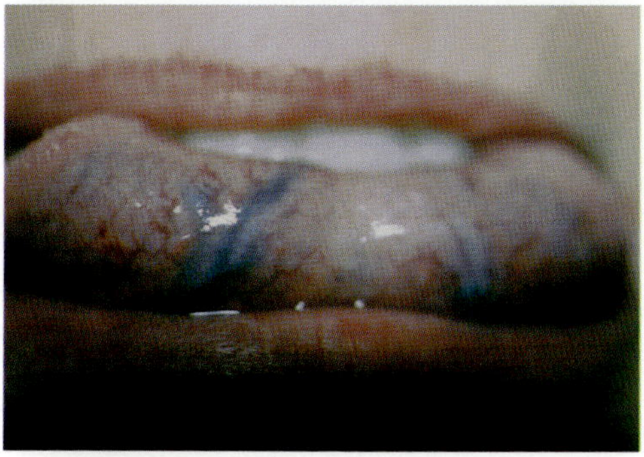

7b

Deep, blue protruding, branch veins on the underside of the tongue:
Liver circulation problems; dark/red spots for heavy metal.

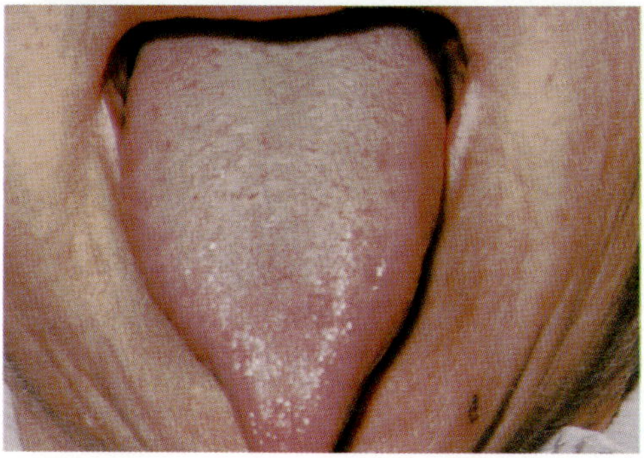

7c

Tip of tongue elongated:
Heart disease.

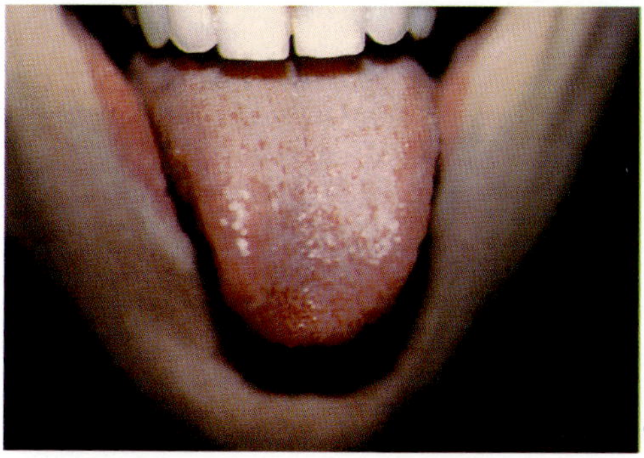

7d

Red spots on the tip of the tongue:
Heart problems, nervousness Insomnia, or thyroid problems.

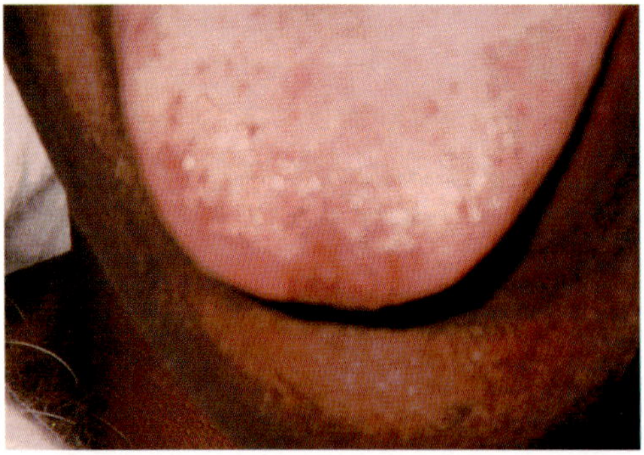

Tip of tongue dark / red:
Heart discase.
(if not a birthmark)

8a

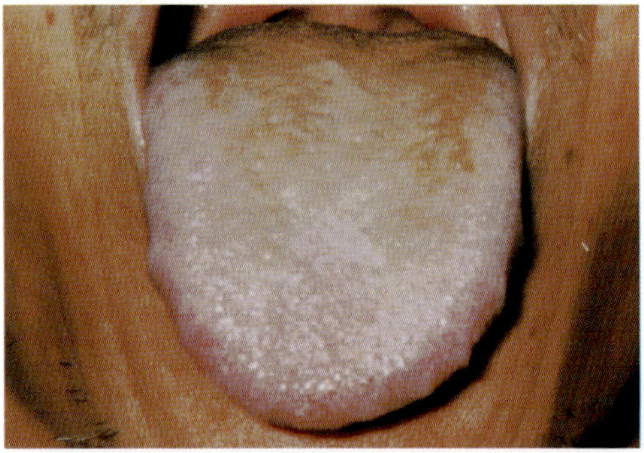

Pulmonary heart problems due to Tuberculosis smoking, poor digestion; spleen/kidney also weak.

8b

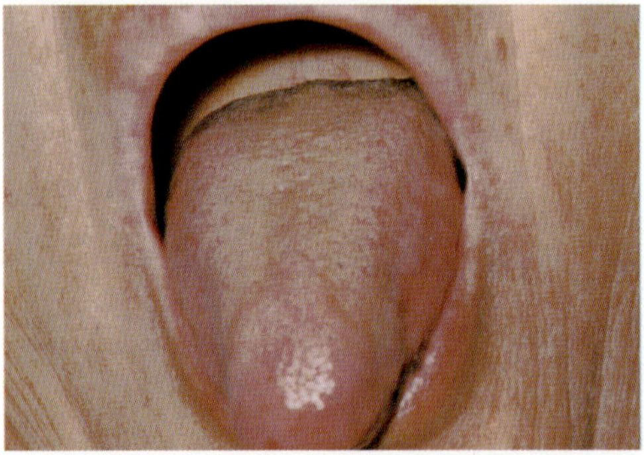

Just over month later from picture 8b with Dr. Chi's remedies can see much improvement.

8c

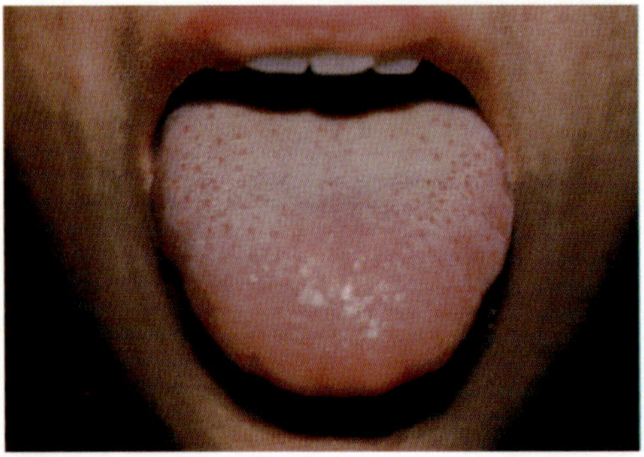

Star- shaped spots:
Hormonal imbalance.

8d

INDEX

Corrections: In the first paragraph on page 31, the figure represented should be Fig. 2-b, not Fig. 1-f. On page 44, Figure 1-f should read "side view, clubbing," instead of "spoon-like." We apologize for any inconvenience caused by these mistakes.